Side Eff

of

Psychiatric Medications

Prevention, Assessment, and Management

(Second edition)

Rajnish Mago, MD

Editor-in-Chief

Simple and Practical Medical Education

(simpleandpractical.com)

ISBN: 9798686376243

CONTENTS

Praise for the First edition

Disclaimer

1 General principles

What's the big deal?

Knowledge is power

Sensitive to medications

2 Anticholinergic side effects

3 Cardiovascular System

Bleeding

Blood pressure

Dizziness (Orthostatic hypotension)

Myocarditis

Q-T prolongation

4 Discontinuation syndromes

Antidepressant discontinuation

Dopamine agonist withdrawal syndrome
(DAWS)

5 Ears

Tinnitus

6 Electrolytes

Hyponatremia

Metabolic acidosis

7 Endocrine glands

Diabetes insipidus (see Polyuria/Diabetes

insipidus)

Hyperparathyroidism

Hyperprolactinemia

Thyroid dysfunction

8   Eyes

Blurred vision

Glaucoma

9   Gastrointestinal tract

Constipation

Diarrhea

Loss of appetite (Anorexia)

Nausea

Pancreatitis

10   Genitals/Sexuality

Sexual dysfunction

11   Blood sugar

Hyperglycemia

12   Liver

Hyperammonemia (elevated serum ammonia level)

13   Mouth

Bruxism

Dry mouth (Xerostomia)

Hypersalivation (Sialorrhea)

14   Nervous system

Akathisia

Headache

Insomnia (see Sleep)

Parkinsonism

Seizures

Tardive dyskinesia

Tremors

Sexuality (see Genitals/sexuality)

15   **Skin**

Acne

Excessive sweating (Hyperhidrosis)

Hair loss (Alopecia)

Skin reactions

16   **Sleep**

Insomnia

17   **Urinary System**

Kidney Stones

Polyuria/Polydipsia

Urinary hesitancy/retention

18   **Weight**

Weight gain

Weight loss (see Loss of Appetite)

19   **Other side effects**

Edema

Yawning

Praise for the First Edition

"Here is one of those gems that one stumbles upon in the clinical literature that warrants much more attention. Dr. Mago's book is concise, practical, and clearly written by someone who recognizes the importance of sensitively addressing side effects and shows clinicians exactly how to do it. The book is suffused with an empathetic understanding of the legitimate concerns side effects have for patients. It is an excellent resource for anyone prescribing psychotropic medications. Indeed, I would highly recommend this succinct, well-crafted book for any clinician's bookshelf, where it will provide practical information for use on a daily basis."

- Shawn Christopher Shea, MD (author of *Psychiatric Interviewing: The Art of Understanding*)

"I believe this book is so useful that it should be required reading for trainees and practitioners as well."

- Harry Croft, MD (author of *I Always Sit with My Back to the Wall: Managing Traumatic Stress and Combat PTSD*)

"The book is as its author's description: simple & practical. It deals with common adverse effects of psychotropics in a simple outline."

- Ahmed Elaghoury, MD

"There are plenty of "academic" books. Some of them are superb, some of them are just wasted money. What [are] scarce are books with clinical pearls and tips. This book [is] filled with them. I found a lot of interesting things and facts that are not discussed in a typical textbook. Not sure if I'll be able to use them all, but at least three tips seem to be very helpful to me. Price is very modest, so I strongly recommend to buy the book."

- Taras Matiiash, MD

"If you prescribe psych meds, this book is for you"

- Marjorie DeStefano, NP

"The book is concise, well written, and pragmatic.

- Jaswinderjit Singh, MD

"This book is a gem. It highlights the importance of being vigilant of side effects and has practical tips about patient education and side effect management."

- Pamela Kaw, MD

"Excellent book covering common side effects of most types of psychotropic medications. Easy to read and informative with strategies about how to treat them."

- David M. Davis, MD

"This is a highly practical, user-friendly, brief book. It is chock full of great tips to use in managing side effects for patients on psychiatric medications."

- Elisabeth Kunkel, MD

Disclaimer

The information in this book is provided for informational and educational purposes for healthcare professionals only, and **not** for patients or other laypersons. It is the responsibility of the prescribing clinicians to evaluate their patients and use their clinical judgment in treating each individual patient.

The contents of this book are **not** intended as medical advice. This information provided is **not** intended to create any physician-patient relationship and is **not** a substitute for professional advice from a licensed healthcare practitioner. It is very important that patients consult their prescribing clinician about any side effects they have and not implement any of the suggestions in this book unless their clinician recommends that they do so.

CHAPTER 1: GENERAL PRINCIPLES

WHAT'S THE BIG DEAL?

Why adverse effects are so important

Adverse effects are more common than we generally think

Clinicians have been heard to say about particular medications that, "Most patients don't have any side effects with it." That is a misleading statement. In fact, adverse effects are common with most or all of the medications we prescribe. In one study of patients taking an SSRI, 52% of patients reported having three or more adverse effects from the SSRI. Thankfully, most of these adverse effects are not medically serious and do not persist long term, but they do cause distress to patients and lead to non-adherence.

Adverse effects cause suffering – sometimes a little, sometimes a lot

OK, time to practice our empathy skills. You have had nausea, haven't you? Imagine taking a medication that causes you to feel nauseous for a couple of hours after each dose. Or makes you put on 20 pounds. Or prevents you from being able to get an erection or have an orgasm. Or makes you extremely self-conscious in public because everyone can see that your hands are shaking. Of patients taking an SSRI, in one study 55% reported having an adverse effect that was moderately or extremely bothersome. For some unfortunate patients, the adverse effects of their medications can be (almost) as bad as the illness itself.

Adverse effects are one of the main reasons that patients stop taking their medications

Do you know what the biggest problem in psychopharmacology is? It is that the majority of patients prematurely stop taking their medications. The reasons for this are complex, but one of the most important reasons for non-adherence to psychiatric medications is occurrence of adverse effects.

By the way, it is important to know specifically WHICH adverse effects of a particular medication are associated with the patient stopping that medication. Why? Because then we can be more sensitive to educating patients about THOSE particular adverse events, preventing (when possible), identifying, and managing those adverse effects aggressively.

How are adverse effects assessed and managed in clinical practice?

Patients will frequently not tell the prescribing clinician about adverse effects they have. Of patients who had side effects attributed by them to an SSRI, 46% reported that they had not discussed these with their physician. Asking a patient a general, open-ended question about any side effects tends to have low sensitivity and specificity. That is, on the one hand, many side effects are missed, and on the other hand, many symptoms that are reported are not really side effects. Perhaps surprisingly, many of the side effects that are missed by open-ended questions are clinically significant — causing functional impairment or requiring some action on the part of the clinician.

How are adverse effects assessed in clinical trials?

You will be surprised to know that in published clinical trials of antidepressants, 86% of the studies did not use any rating scale or specific method for identification of adverse effects; instead, they relied only on "spontaneous reporting."

KNOWLEDGE IS POWER

Effective strategies for educating patients about potential

adverse effects

Why is this a problem?

There are several reasons why educating patients about adverse effects is challenging. If we were to ask several prescribing clinicians what the potential adverse effects of a particular medication are, they would list only a few of the common ones and would disagree considerably. Unless a specific strategy is used, trying to resolve this by looking at the Physician's Desk Reference or the Prescribing Information is likely to make one's eyes glaze over because of the very long list of potential adverse events, many with dubious relationship to the medication.

If a patient asks, "Doctor, what are the side effects that could occur with this medication?" it is surprising that a straight answer to this simple question is not readily available. Try it – what are the common adverse effects of escitalopram, venlafaxine, zolpidem, or divalproex? Compare your answers to the lists provided in the Appendix.

Ok, what's the plan, then?

Let us start by defining our goals: we want to tell our patients about common side effects, not to give them a comprehensive list that includes problems that might occur in < 1% of patients. In addition, we want to tell them about adverse effects that may be particularly dangerous, even if they are not common.

But what does it mean to call an adverse effect "common." Let's agree on the following cut offs that are sometimes used: we will call an adverse effect "common" if it occurs in 5% or more of patients on that medication. We will call an adverse effect "less common" if it occurs in at least 1% but less than 5% of patients on that medication. Adverse effects that occur in less than 1% of patients we will call "uncommon" and we will not routinely tell patients about them (unless they are particular important due to being dangerous, as discussed below).

But wait — how do we know if a symptom that occurs with a medication is, in fact, an adverse effect of the medication? That opens a whole other can of worms, so let's just say that if the symptom occurs at least twice as often on the medication than on placebo, we will assume that it is related to the medication.

This then brings up one last question: should we tell the patient how often the problem occurred in patients on the medication OR how often it occurred in patients on the medication AND could be attributed to the medication? For example, if a problem occurred in 7% of patients on the medication and 2% of patients on placebo, should we tell the patient it occurs in 7% of patients or in 5% of patients (7 minus 2)? This is a hard one. Until we come up with a better answer, it may be best to tell the patient both numbers and say that the problem occurred in 7% of patients on the medication and would be attributed to the medication in 5% of patients.

Since it is unacceptable that our patients not get a straight answer —in writing— a handout specific to each drug has been prepared and is included in the Appendix to this book.

How to document education about adverse effects

First, let us see what is not an optimum approach. Trying to list all the adverse effects you told the patient would be too time consuming. Listing a limited number of adverse effects may be worse because in effect you may be documenting that you did NOT tell the patient about certain other potential adverse effects. Having the patient sign a prepared list of adverse effects that they were told about can be problematic if the number of adverse effects is limited or, conversely, if it is exhaustive. Courts are not impressed with a document, signed by a patient, that includes (in small print) dozens of potential adverse effects.

One option is to document "Risks discussed, consent obtained" or "RDCO" and "handouts given." We must attach copies of the handouts given to the patient that list the common adverse effects and the potentially dangerous adverse effects that the patient was told about. It is important to attach a copy of the exact handout that was given since the handout you use in your practice may change over time. If the prescriber has documented this education, it is probably not essential that the patient sign a document acknowledging receipt of the handouts.

What if there was a simple thing you could do that could significantly reduce the number of patients who stop taking the medications that you prescribe? The frustrating thing is that the great majority of patients stop their medication soon after starting it, not because of a serious adverse event, but due to something that is not medically dangerous. If we tell our patients the following five things when starting a new medication, we can significantly reduce this.

1. Most side effects of the medication are "Nuisance side effects" rather than "Medically serious side effects." They are definitely bothersome and we will do something about them, but it is important for you to know that these nuisance side effects will not harm any organ of your body.

2. Most side effects occur during the first 30 days, while the medication may be taken for many months or years. If we can work together to get through the first 30 days, very few new side effects are likely to come up.

3. Most of these side effects diminish within a few days or weeks.

4. For many side effects, there is something we can do to help reduce the side effect.

5. So, if any symptoms occur that you think may be side effects of the medication, don't stop taking the medication. Call me and we'll together decide what we should do.

SENSITIVE TO MEDICATIONS

Assessment

All prescribing clinicians periodically encounter persons who seem to have an unusually higher severity of adverse effects from medications. They describe themselves as being "sensitive to medications" and tend to have side effects on relatively low doses of medications.

I am sure you have seen some patients like this, right? This situation can be very frustrating for both the patient and the clinician.

Important! The ability to treat patients who are sensitive to one or more medications is essential for anyone who wants to be considered an "expert" psychopharmacologist.

1.   Does the patient have panic disorder?

Patients with panic disorder are often particularly sensitive to adverse effects of medications. This may be, at least in part, to their higher degree of somatic sensitivity. That is, any side effects that they have may be experienced by them with higher intensity.

2. Is the patient quite anxious?

It has been observed in clinical experience and also formally shown that patients who are significantly anxious tend to experience more adverse effects.

3. Could a drug-drug interaction be causing higher drug levels?

The possibility of drug-drug interactions should always be kept in mind when there is either low response or higher adverse effects. I strongly recommend that we should not just rely on our own fund of knowledge about drug-drug interactions. In all patients, a drug interaction search should be performed.

For doing a quick drug interaction search, I like using online.epocrates.com that is free, quick, and provides only brief information rather than lengthy explanations that would take a while to read. For how to do this in less than one minute, see How to do a drug interaction search in one minute.

4. Genetically lower metabolism of the medication?

Could the patient have a genetic polymorphism of the cytochrome P450 system that makes him or her a poor metabolizer of the drug, leading to higher drug levels?

Testing for such polymorphisms is now clinically available and should be strongly considered in patients who have unexpectedly greater side effects on a medication that is metabolized by those specific isoenzymes. I have seen many patients who had unexpected side effects and turned out to be poor metabolizers on the exact isoenzyme that metabolizes that particular medication.

My own research showed that for selected antidepressants, about 2/3rds of patients who had a higher number/ intensity of side effects were poor/ intermediate metabolizers on the CYP450 isoenzymes that metabolize those antidepressants.

To interpret such testing, we need to know which medications are metabolized by which P450 isoenzymes. See Which CYP 450 isoenzyme metabolizes which medication?

5. <u>Does the patient have difficulty trusting caregivers?</u>

Was the patient abused or betrayed by caregivers in the past? Patients who have had such experiences, may perceive treatments as being harmful even when they are not.

6. <u>Does the patient have negative views of medications in general?</u>

It is, unfortunately, common for patients to believe that medications are harmful and should be avoided. One clue to this is when a patient refers to the medication as "the drug." Or, instead of talking about "taking the medication," refers to "putting it in my body." If we listen to our patients carefullly, we can become aware of these things.

Management

1. All patients with panic disorder should always be started on half (or even less than half) of usual doses of medications, e.g., antidepressants.

2. When a drug-drug interaction is present, in some cases, a different medication can be chosen. We often assume that this has to be a different psychotropic medication, but depending on the situation, it could be the non-psychiatric medication that is changed to avoid the drug-drug interaction.

3. In other cases, the drug-drug interaction that is raising the levels of the psychotropic medication can be taken into account by both starting with a lower than usual dose and maintaining the patient on a lower than usual dose.

4. When a psychotropic medication is continued at a lower dose because the patient is also taking the drug that raises the levels of the psychotropic, keep in mind that the dose of the psychotropic medication will also have to be adjusted if the offending agent is stopped. Often, the drug-drug interaction is missed at the "back end."

5. Whenever possible, drug levels should be obtained to guide the dosing of the medication.

6. When a patient who is quite anxious requires a medication like an antidepressant, it can be helpful to first reduce the anxiety over a few days by prescribing a benzodiazepine and only then starting the antidepressant.

7. I have successfully managed many patients who are very sensitive to medications by starting them on very small doses. For example, sertraline can be started at 12.5 mg/day by prescribing half of a 25 mg pill. Low doses of medications can also be given more conveniently by using liquid formulations of medications. The overall dose of the medication can also be lowered by taking it on alternate days or even less frequently than that.

8. Extreme problems sometimes require extreme measures. For patients who are exquisitely sensitive to medications, sometimes I start the patient on ridiculously small doses. For example, I ask the patient to start by crushing the pill (for pills that are not sustained-release preparations). This can be done by buying and using a pill crusher, or more simply by wrapping the pill in a clean sheet of paper and crushing it with a spoon or a hammer. Then, I ask the patient to start with the smallest grain of the crushed pill that is possible. I know — this is extreme, but I have been able to help many patients by using this approach when they have failed treatment with several other physicians.

9.   When patients start on lower than usual doses, they can sometimes progress gradually to usual doses but in some cases will benefit from and continue on lower than usual doses. There are probably many different reasons, some known and some unknown, why patients have different blood levels of medications, and different degrees of response and adverse effects with the same blood levels. In the end, we must treat the patient based on the individual patient's response and not insist on prescribing the usual recommended dose.

10. Since psychological factors can either help or hinder the patient's ability to tolerate the medication, I believe it is psychologically extremely important that the patient be told clearly and emphatically that the dose being prescribed is infinitesimally low. Sometimes I tell the patient that the dose I am giving them is more suitable for a newborn baby than for an adult. This usually helps significantly in reducing the patient's anxiety about the medication.

11. Similarly, in my experience it is extremely helpful when titrating up from very low doses to emphasize to the patient that only when the patient feels comfortable with a dose and thinks she would be OK with trying a slightly higher dose should the dose be increased. This will prevent the patient from fearing that she might be pressured to increase the dose before being ready to do so. Giving the patient a measure of control over the dose titration helps to reduce this anxiety.

References: See https://simpleandpractical.com/side-effects-references

CHAPTER 2: ANTICHOLINERGIC SIDE EFFECTS

Clinical case: New onset of acute anxiety and physical symptoms

Clinical vignette: A patient's primary care physician had recently put her on two medications to treat her irritable bowel syndrome:

– Dicyclomine (brand name Bentyl) 20 mg three times a day

– Hyoscyamine 0.125 mg four times a day.

After a week or so of taking the medications, the patient began to develop anxiety, which soon became quite intense. She also had several physical symptoms—a racing heart, flushed face, worsening constipation, extreme thirst, dry mouth, feeling very hot, and urinary retention.

The patient decided, on her own, to stop the medications. Her anxiety and physical symptoms subsided rapidly after the medications were stopped.

What do you think had happened to this patient?

Dicyclomine and hyoscyamine are both anticholinergic medications. Our colleague diagnosed the patient as having had anticholinergic toxicity from simultaneously starting two anticholinergic medications at full doses. The patient was relieved to hear there was an explanation for her symptoms and was grateful for this. Since the symptoms had resolved and there was no history of anxiety except during the anticholinergic toxicity, no psychiatric treatment was recommended.

How does toxicity from anticholinergic medications present clinically?

Many medications have anticholinergic properties and anticholinergic toxicity is very common in the US.

Here is a mnemonic that helps us to remember the clinical features of anticholinergic toxicity (Broderick et al., 2020).

"Red as a beet, dry as a bone, blind as a bat, mad as a hatter, hot as a hare, full as a flask."

"Red as a beet": Flushing of the skin. Since anticholinergic activity blocks sweating, blood vessels in the skin dilate so that heat loss from the skin can be increased. This is the same principle that explains why we get red in the face when we are in a hot environment.

"Dry as a bone": Lack of sweating (anhidrosis), dry mucous membranes

"Blind as a bat": Blurred vision due to blocking of accommodation and dilation of the pupils (mydriasis)

"Mad as a hatter": Confusion, disorientation, anxiety, agitation, hallucinations, persecutory delusions, etc. This is why the patient may be thought to have a primary psychiatric problem.

"Hot as a hare": Fever; this also occurs because anticholinergic activity blocks sweating and, so, heat loss.

"Full as a flask": Urinary retention

There are two common and important symptoms that are not covered by this famous mnemonic:

– Tachycardia

– Decreased bowel sounds

Also, it is important for us to know that anticholinergic toxicity can also lead to prolongation of the QTc interval.

In older adults, avoid medications with anticholinergic activity

We know that cholinergic activity is important for memory and cognition, right? Anticholinergic medications can cause cognitive impairment. On the other hand, cholinesterase inhibitors that reduce breakdown of acetylcholine (e.g., donepezil, galantamine, rivastigmine) are used for the treatment of Alzheimer's disease and other dementias.

But it is not only "anticholinergic medications" like benztropine, trihexyphenidyl, etc that have anticholinergic activity. Several other psychotropic and non-psychotropic medications also have high or moderate levels of anticholinergic activity.

In any person, especially an older adult, who presents with cognitive impairment (including dementia), the list of the person's medications should be reviewed to identify medications that have significant anticholinergic activity.

How common is use of medications with anticholinergic activity?

We may think that use in older adults of medications with significant anticholinergic activity is relatively rare. Apparently not.

1. General population

About 10% of older adults in the US are taking a potentially inappropriate medication with significant anticholinergic activity (Kachru et al., 2015).

2. Persons with cognitive impairment

Even more concerning, it is common even for patients attending a memory clinic to be taking a medication with anticholinergic activity (Barton et al., 2008). In fact, some such patients were found to be taking both a cholinesterase inhibitor and a medication with anticholinergic properties (Barton et al., 2008)!

Of persons with dementia, 27% were found to be taking a potentially inappropriate medication with significant anticholinergic activity (Kachru et al., 2003).

Which medications have significant anticholinergic activity?

We can assume that the reason that many older adults get medications with anticholinergic activity is because the prescribing clinician was not aware that the medication had significant anticholinergic activity.

Here are the most frequently prescribed medications (psychotropic and non-psychotropic) with significant anticholinergic activity (Kachru et al., 2003; Barton et al., 2008; Kachru et al., 2015). Let's try to avoid these medications in elderly patients whenever possible. Let's also look for them as possible causes in any patient with cognitive impairment. They are listed here alphabetically.

<u>Antidepressants</u>

Amitriptyline

Paroxetine

<u>Antihistamines</u>

e.g.,

Diphenhydramine (Benadryl®)

Hydroxyzine (Atarax®, Vistaril®)

Promethazine (Phenargan®)

<u>Antispasmodics</u>

e.g.,

Dicyclomine (Bentyl®)

<u>Medications for overactive bladder</u>

e.g.,

Oxybutynin (Ditropan®)

Solifenacin (Vesicare®)

Tolterodine (Detrol®)

<u>Other</u>

Cyclobenzaprine (Flexeril®; used for the treatment of muscle stiffness and spasms)

In addition to these more commonly prescribed medications, there are many other medications that are that have high or moderate anticholinergic activity (e.g., doxepin, nortriptyline, olanzapine, quetiapine). Therefore, in a person presenting with cognitive impairment, the person's list of medications should be checked against a comprehensive list of medications with significant anticholinergic activity.

Are doxepin's anticholinergic effects dose-dependent?

Question: Are [the anticholinergic effects of doxepin] dose-dependent? For example, would doxepin 3 to 10 mg as prescribed for sleep be as harmful as doxepin as prescribed for depression?

At higher doses

Doxepin is well-known to be associated with clinically-significant anticholinergic effects like dry mouth, constipation, memory impairment, tachycardia, urinary hesitancy or retention, and so on (Chew et al., 2008; Feighner et al., 1986; Feighner and Cohn, 1985; Arnold et al., 1981).

At low doses

But, what about at low doses?

Clinical trials of low-dose doxepin (1 mg, 3 mg, 6 mg) in adults (Krystal et al., 2011; Roth et al., 2007) or even specifically in elderly adults (Lankford et al., 2012; Krystal et al., 2010; Scharf et al., 2008) did not find any reports of anticholinergic side effects like dry mouth, memory impairment, etc. A limitation of these data is that clinical trials don't specifically and actively look for these side effects; they rely on patients to spontaneously report any adverse events (Mago, 2016).

But, the Prescribing Information for low-dose doxepin (brand name Silenor) notes that dry mouth, constipation, etc. have been infrequently or rarely reported in patients on low-dose doxepin.

Bottom line

We can conclude, in answering our question, that, yes, the anticholinergic side effects of doxepin are dose-dependent.

At low doses of up to 6 mg per day, doxepin is not associated with any clinically-relevant anticholinergic effects (Richey and Krystal, 2011).

Despite this, we should remember that, in elderly patients, the recommended starting dose of doxepin is 3 mg per day (Prescribing Information).

Use a rating scale for anticholinergic burden from medications

In any person, especially an older adult, who presents with cognitive impairment (including dementia), the list of the person's medications should be systematically reviewed to identify medications that have significant anticholinergic activity.

In most cases, a high anticholinergic burden is due to the cumulative effect of multiple medications that individually have low anticholinergic potency rather than due to a single high potency anticholinergic medication (Mate et al., 2015), a fact that is often not considered when prescribing medications.

It is not enough to know a few of the commonly used drugs that possess anticholinergic activity. Instead, just like the Flockhart table for CYP450 interactions, it is critical to use one of the rating scales for anticholinergic activity since so many psychotropic and non-psychotropic medications have anticholinergic properties and it is such an important issue in older adults.

To do this, thankfully we don't need to memorize all the medications that have significant anticholinergic activity. Various "scales" are available that we can refer to.

Examples of these are Anticholinergic Cognitive Burden scale (Boustani et al., 2008), Anticholinergic Drug Scale, Anticholinergic Risk Scale (Rudolph et al., 2008), Drug Burden Index—Anticholinergic component (DBI-ACh), etc.

For day-to-day clinical use, I recommend using the Anticholinergic Cognitive Burden (ACB) Scale (Boustani et al., 2008) which can be found HERE. I like the Anticholinergic Cognitive Burden (ACB) Scale as it is just the right length. The Anticholinergic Risk Scale covers too few medications and other lists are very long (e.g., Duran et al., 2013).

I have the Anticholinergic Cognitive Burden (ACB) Scale on my clipboard along with a couple of other useful tools. This scale can be used to score each medication that the person is taking as zero (no

23

anticholinergic activity) or on a three-point scale. The points are then added up to give a total score that reflects the total anticholinergic burden of the medications that the person is taking.

I then send a report to the primary care physician, saying something like "in this patient who presents with cognitive impairment, the anticholinergic burden is fairly high with 5 medications contributing to a total score of 14. Every attempt should be made to replace these medications with non-anticholinergic alternatives (and I will make specific recommendations here), as this may significantly improve cognitive functioning. Please do not hesitate to contact me if there are any concerns about these recommendations".

A score looks more impressive and definitive than a vague general statement, and primary care physicians are used to scoring everything so it fits in well with their worldview.

I then recommend repeating cognitive screening in 4 to 6 months. Improvement in cognitive functioning does not correspond to the half-life of the medications but lags way behind, often by many months. Except for the most severe cases, I try to hold off on making a formal diagnosis of dementia until then. I have seen even MoCA scores as low as 16 normalize once the anticholinergic medications were removed.

The biggest problem is in getting any buy-in from the primary care physicians. Sometimes I see patients back in my office a few months later and none of the medications have been replaced. Changing 3 to 5 medications can take more time than a busy primary care physician has in 1 or 2 office visits. Also, some of the medications may have been prescribed not by the primary care physician but by another specialist. Patience and active communication with the primary care physician are needed in such cases. When the primary care physicians see in one or two of their patients what an improvement the recommended medication changes can make, they really start to take an interest in reducing the anticholinergic burden of medications.

References: See https://simpleandpractical.com/side-effects-references

CHAPTER 3: CARDIOVASCULAR SYSTEM

BLEEDING

How do antidepressants increase the risk of bleeding?

If case you are thinking—*How is this "practical"?*—understanding the mechanisms by which antidepressants increase the risk of bleeding will tell us which antidepressants to use in persons who are at higher risk of bleeding and what else we can do to reduce the risk of bleeding.. So, stay with me!

Inhibition of serotonin uptake on platelets

The main, though maybe not only, mechanism by which some antidepressants increase the risk of bleeding is the same as that by antidepressants like SSRIs work—inhibition of serotonin uptake.

Remember that platelets stop bleeding by clumping together and forming a platelet plug? This clumping is triggered by the release of serotonin from platelets in response to injury (Li et al., 1997). Amazingly, the platelet reuptake site on platelets is the exact same molecule as the serotonin transporter on serotonergic neurons in the brain (Lesch et al., 1993).

Serotonin reuptake inhibitor antidepressants (SSRIs, SNRIs, and some others) significantly inhibit the uptake of serotonin into platelets (Hergovich et al., 2000). Since platelets don't make serotonin, their serotonin content goes down a lot when a serotonin reuptake inhibitor antidepressant is given. This depletion of serotonin leads to impairment in the ability of platelets to stop bleeding.

Inhibition of platelet function by other mechanisms

[Optional to read: In addition to inhibition of serotonin uptake, other mechanisms may also be involved in how some antidepressants inhibit platelet aggregation (e.g., Roweth et al., 2011).]

Increase in the secretion of gastric acid

Given that bleeding related to antidepressant use is most likely to be gastrointestinal, it is important that, in addition to inhibiting platelet aggregation, some antidepressants also increase the secretion of gastric acid (Andrade et al., 2010). This also has practical importance because it is believed that using a proton pump inhibitor reduces the risk of gastrointestinal bleeding associated with antidepressant use.

Antidepressants and bleeding: What are the high risk factors?

Serotonergic antidepressants are associated with an increased risk of bleeding. This is because they inhibit the aggregation of platelets.

How can we anticipate this problem by identifying high-risk factors?

Important: This risk of bleeding becomes much more if more than one risk factor is present.

Patients at higher risk of bleeding are:

1. Older adults

2. Have hepatitis C (Weinrieb et al., 2003).

Let's keep in mind that SSRIs are often prescribed for the treatment of interferon-induced depression in these patients. If the patient has cirrhosis/ portal hypertension, there is an increased risk of GI bleeding, though only a very small percentage of patients may have such bleeding (e.g., Martin et al., 2007).

3. Taking aspirin or NSAIDs

The risk of gastrointestinal bleeding in a person who is taking an SSRI is nearly 4 times that of the general population. But if the person is taking both an SSRI and an NSAID, the risk is 12 times that of the general population.

4. Taking antiplatelet medications

E.g., heparin, clopidogrel (Plavix®; e.g., Labos et al., 2011).

5. Taking over-the-counter medications that affect clotting

E.g., vitamin E, fish oil

Are some SSRIs associated with a lesser or greater risk of bleeding?

Avoid antidepressants with a high affinity for the serotonin transporter?

Based on our understanding, discussed above, of why antidepressants may lead to an increased risk of bleeding, one might think that the increased risk of bleeding with antidepressants would be directly correlated with the extent to which the antidepressant inhibits serotonin uptake by platelets.

As we discussed earlier, the serotonin uptake site on platelets is the same as the serotonin reuptake site on presynaptic neurons. So, we can assume that the affinity of antidepressants for serotonin uptake sites on platelets and presynaptic neurons will be the same.

High affinity (alphabetically): clomipramine, fluoxetine, paroxetine, sertraline.

Moderate affinity (alphabetically): amitriptyline, citalopram, escitalopram, fluvoxamine, imipramine, venlafaxine, vilazodone, vortioxetine.

Low or no affinity (alphabetically): agomelatine, amoxapine, bupropion, desipramine, doxepin, maprotiline, mianserin, mirtazapine, moclobemide, nefazodone, nortriptyline, reboxetine, trazodone, trimipramine.

Bottom line

We are not completely sure but it seems that antidepressants with a higher affinity for the serotonin transporter—clomipramine, fluoxetine, paroxetine, sertraline—may be more likely to increase the risk of bleeding than other antidepressants.

Are antidepressants that don't inhibit serotonin uptake less likely to increase the risk of bleeding?

This is a clinically important question:

When patients are at increased risk of bleeding (e.g., on chronic NSAID or anticoagulation treatment, history of bleeding) and need an antidepressant, are there particular antidepressants that may be safer?

The hypothesis

As we discussed above, the main mechanism by which antidepressants increase the risk of bleeding is inhibition of serotonin uptake by platelets leading to decreased clumping (aggregation) of platelets to form a platelet plug in response to injury. So, one would expect that antidepressants that do not inhibit serotonin uptake (like bupropion, mirtazapine, reboxetine, agomelatine, and so on) would be less likely to increase the risk of bleeding, right?

The current state of knowledge

Some studies found an increased risk of bleeding with serotonin reuptake inhibitors but not with other antidepressants (e.g., Meijer et al., 2004; de Abajo et al., 2008). But, a meta-analysis of studies did not find the risk of bleeding to be statistically significantly lower with antidepressants like mirtazapine and bupropion compared to serotonin reuptake inhibitors (Na et al., 2018). The studies have many limitations that I won't get into here. But, I want to make a few points in this regard:

1. We should not think that the studies show that the increased risk of bleeding is the SAME for serotonin reuptake inhibitors and other antidepressants. To show that the risk is the same would require much larger sample sizes and a different type of statistical approach.

2. What we can say is that the idea that antidepressants like mirtazapine and bupropion are not associated with as much of an increased risk of bleeding as serotonin reuptake inhibitors has not been clearly shown yet.

3. Also, even if the extent of increased risk is less with these antidepressants, it may not be zero. This is because it is possible that mechanisms other than inhibition of serotonin uptake may be operating.

[Optional to read: A case report of epistaxis associated with mirtazapine use has been published (Mirza and Majeed, 2018), but this is not convincing evidence of an increased risk of bleeding with the use of mirtazapine.]

[Optional to read: One study in rats found that mirtazapine had a protective effect against indomethacin-induced gastric ulcers (Bilici et al., 2009)]

Bottom line

Various authors recommended that antidepressants that do not inhibit serotonin reuptake—like bupropion, mirtazapine, and others—should be preferred in patients who are at increased risk of bleeding (e.g., Mago et al., 2008; Andrade et al., 2010; Sayadipour et al., 2012; Jeong et al., 2014; Bixby et al., 2019).

It makes sense to do this if possible.

Due to possible indirect effects of bupropion and mirtazapine, one paper hypothesized that bupropion may be an even better option than mirtazapine (Na et al., 2018), but this has not been proven yet.

Antidepressants and bleeding: When and what to ask

Serotonergic antidepressants can be associated with an increased tendency to bleed. Thankfully, this is not clinically important in the great majority of patients. But, if a person has certain risk factor(s), the risk of bleeding can increase by more than 10 times.

When should we ask patients who are on a serotonergic antidepressant additional questions?

1. If they have at least one risk factor for an increased tendency to bleed

2. If they show any signs of increased bleeding

I am embarrassed to admit that I have seen several patients who had multiple bruises all over their body and didn't think to relate them to the fact that the person was on a serotonergic antidepressant. Because of that, I have now become good at noticing that a patient has multiple bruises and asking the patient additional questions to follow up on that observation.

3. If the person is going to have elective surgery

Even though most surgeons and even mental health clinicians don't seem to know about this, many studies have shown that some persons who are on a serotonergic antidepressant can have a clinically significant increase in bleeding during surgery.

What should we ask?

1. As in all patients, during the initial evaluation and at each visit, we should make sure we are aware of ALL the medications the person is taking. This includes prescription medications, over-the-counter medications, supplements, and herbal medications. We should be aware of any antiplatelet agents, aspirin or NSAIDs, fish oil, etc. We should also be aware of any drug-drug interactions that may increase the effects of the patient's medications, e.g., antiplatelet agents.

2. In the patients described in the section above, we should ask about early signs of an increased tendency to bleed. What are some "simple and practical" questions that we can ask for this?

– Easy bruising, e.g., after a minor bump

– Bleeding for longer than expected after getting blood drawn for laboratory tests

– Bleeding for longer than expected after a cut while shaving (or any other injury)

– New onset of bleeding after flossing

Antidepressants and risk of stroke

We have long known that use of an antidepressant along with an NSAID increases risk of gastrointestinal bleeding. I always prescribe a proton pump inhibitor in patients who are taking both types of medications.

However, what can we do to reduce the risk of intracranial hemorrhage in patients who take an antidepressant and an NSAID together?

1. Rethink as to whether or not each of these medications — the antidepressant and the NSAID — are absolutely essential. If not, consider stopping one of them.

2. If an antidepressant is essential in a patient taking an NSAID, strongly consider using a medication with little or no serotonergic activity, e.g., bupropion.

3. Consider platelet function testing (NOT prothrombin time or partial thromboplastin time) to assess the degree to which the medications are affecting platelet function.

DIZZINESS (ORTHOSTATIC HYPOTENSION)

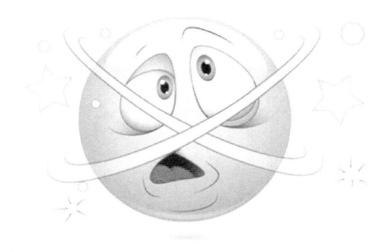

Orthostatic hypotension/ dizziness is a (potentially) serious adverse effect

An orthostatic drop in blood pressure can cause a person to fall or even to faint. It should always be taken seriously. It is not rare for a patient, especially one who is older, to faint or fall due to medication-induced orthostatic dizziness and to sustain significant injuries. Are we doing enough to reduce falls?

Our meds are often the cause!

Many psychotropic medications can cause orthostatic hypotension including second-generation antipsychotics (especially risperidone and clozapine), tricyclic antidepressants, trazodone, benzodiazepines, and monoamine oxidase inhibitors (MAOIs). Therefore, prescribers of psychotropic medications must know how to evaluate and manage orthostatic hypotension.

What causes orthostatic hypotension?

First a simple and quick reminder about why orthostatic hypotension occurs. Normally, when a person rises up from a lying down or sitting position, and blood pools in the legs, a drop in blood pressure is recognized by baroreceptors (pressure receptors) in the aorta and elsewhere. This triggers a reflex that causes the blood vessels to constrict which in turn keeps the blood pressure up. Since the receptors on the blood vessels – through which this reflex occurs – are alpha-1 receptors, any medication that blocks alpha-1 receptors reduces this compensatory response. With such medications, when the patient rises from a lying down or seated position, the blood pressure temporarily drops, which is called orthostatic (literally, "in the straight position") or postural hypotension. Blood flow to the head decreases and the person feels dizzy.

As noted above, medications that block alpha-1 receptors can cause orthostatic hypotension. Examples of these include the second-generation antipsychotics, tricyclic antidepressants, trazodone, and monoamine oxidase inhibitors (MAOIs).

What kind of "dizziness"?

Persons with orthostatic hypotension typically report feeling "faint", "lightheaded," or "dizzy". But dizziness can mean two completely different things:

1. An orthostatic drop in blood pressure usually leads to a sense of faintness, of dark coming over the eyes, or of feeling "woozy."

2. If objects look like they are spinning, that is vertigo and may be due to inner ear disease.

However, more recent studies have shown that persons with orthostatic hypotension can present not only with lightheadedness, but also with vertigo (Kim et al., 2015). If the person presents with vertigo and orthostatic hypotension is not found to be the explanation, the person should be referred to an ENT doctor.

What other symptoms to ask for

Dizziness is not the only symptom of orthostatic hypotension. We should ask for these other symptoms too:

These may include vague uneasiness, visual disturbances (dimness, blurring, or tunnel vision), vertigo, palpitations, pressure in the head, anxiety, symptoms of sympathetic activation (shakiness, feeling clammy), or syncope (Kim et al., 2015). Sometimes, a dull pain in the back of the neck and shoulder (coat hanger distribution) is described (Shibao et al., 2013).

We should also ask when the symptoms are worse. This is better than asking a leading question about whether the dizziness is worse on standing up. If the dizziness is worse on standing up from a lying, sitting, or bent over position, it is said to be "orthostatic". Typically, the symptoms don't occur when the person is lying down and get better when the person sits down or lies down (Shibao et al., 2013).

A simple thing to do in our office

Have the patient rapidly stand up in our presence (while you are ready to catch the patient if she starts to fall) to see if the subjective complaint is reproduced by a change in posture. By doing this in our office, we also get an idea about how significant the problem is.

Note: if the person has no symptoms but an orthostatic drop in blood pressure is identified by measurement of blood pressure (as described below), this should still be taken seriously because the person is at risk of falls or syncope (Shibao et al., 2013).

Postprandial orthostatic hypotension

This is relatively common in persons with diabetic neuropathy. It is more likely to occur after consuming hot food or drinks, carbohydrates, or alcohol (Figueroa et al., 2010). These patients should be told to reduce their intake of alcohol and to eat in smaller but more frequent meals (Figueroa et al., 2010).

How to correctly measure and interpret orthostatic blood pressure and pulse

Instead of only assessing orthostatic symptoms by history, we must actually measure orthostatic blood pressure and pulse to:

1. Determine whether orthostatic hypotension is really the cause of the symptoms.

2. Determine the severity of the orthostatic hypotension.

3. Determine if the orthostatic hypotension is likely to be neurogenic (see below).

4. Monitor change over time with treatment.

However, a correct method needs to be followed. Have the patient lie down for about 5 minutes. If there is no place for the person to lie down, then have the person sit and rest for 5 minutes. Then, measure the blood pressure and pulse rate. While measurement of the change in blood pressure from sitting to standing may miss some cases of orthostatic hypotension, it is still useful if the setting does not permit measurement of change in blood pressure from lying to standing (Shibao et al., 2013). So, if we can't do the measurement in the ideal way, we should still do what we can!

Next, deflate the blood pressure cuff but leave it on and have the patient stand up. Importantly, have the patient keep standing for one minute, measure the blood pressure and the pulse rate, and then measure again after the person has been standing for three minutes. Measurement at one minute evaluates immediate drop in blood pressure while measurement at three minutes evaluates a slightly delayed drop.

A drop in systolic blood pressure of 20 mmHg or more and/or a drop in diastolic blood pressure of 10 mmHg or more from lying to standing position occurring within 3 minutes has been the standard, accepted definition of orthostatic hypotension for many years. A drop in systolic blood pressure of 20 mmHg or more has been shown to correlate with falls (Shibao et al., 2013).

Some tips:

a) The orthostatic blood pressure tends to vary from time to time, so if the orthostatic blood pressure is normal though suggestive symptoms are present, we should consider repeating the measurement of orthostatic blood pressure. We should especially try to measure it at the time of the day that dizziness or other symptoms occurred (Puisieux et al., 1999).

b) How much of a drop of blood pressure denotes orthostatic hypotension depends in part on what the blood pressure is. So, for a person who is currently hypertensive, a blood pressure drop of 30 mmHg or more may be a more appropriate definition of orthostatic hypotension (Freeman et al., 2011).

c) It is not uncommon for patients with an orthostatic drop of between 10 and 20 mmHg to have clinical symptoms. Also, smaller drops in blood pressure of 10 to 19 mmHg predict greater drops at other times of the day (Weiss et al., 2004). Therefore, I recommend taking a drop in systolic blood pressure of more than 10 mmHg seriously if a clinical picture suggestive of orthostatic hypotension is present. I myself have seen many such patients.

d) Typically, the drop in the blood pressure is accompanied by an increase in the pulse rate as the heart tries to compensate for the drop in blood pressure. It is important that we not forget to also measure the change in pulse rate! If the pulse rate does not increase to compensate for the drop in blood pressure, this usually suggests neurogenic orthostatic hypotension.

Prevent and identify

1. Identify the high-risk patient. Orthostatic hypotension is very common in the elderly (Hitola et al., 2009), especially if the person has low body weight or is frail. Other risk factors include dehydration, diabetes, Parkinson's disease, being on a lot of medications (especially antihypertensives or diuretics). Patients whose blood pressure at baseline is on the low side have lower "reserves" and tend to become symptomatic with smaller orthostatic drops in blood pressure. In addition, orthostatic hypotension can be particularly problematic in patients with significant cardiovascular or cerebrovascular disease. These are the patients in whom we must take preventive measures and whom we must specifically assess for orthostatic hypotension.

In addition, here are some more things to watch out for:

Even a benign infection like a urinary tract infection can markedly worsen orthostatic hypotension (Shibao et al., 2013).

Deconditioning, even just a few days of bed rest (Shibao et al., 2013), as may occur in a person with severe depression.

Orthostatic hypotension tends to be worse in the morning, soon after waking up (Shibao et al., 2013). However, when it is being caused by a medication, it could be worse about 2 hours after taking the medication. We should ask the person to take note of when and under what circumstances the symptoms are worse.

2. Specifically assess. If a higher-risk patient is given a medication that is known to cause orthostatic hypotension, specifically remember to ask the patient about the presence of any orthostatic dizziness. In addition, measure the blood pressure and pulse in the lying and standing position (as described above) at baseline and periodically during treatment.

3. In the predisposed patient, avoid medications that cause orthostatic hypotension when possible. In particular, think about additive effects. In the predisposed patient, avoid using more than one medication that can cause orthostatic hypotension, for example, risperidone along with trazodone for sleep.

How to correctly measure and interpret orthostatic blood pressure and pulse

Instead of only assessing orthostatic symptoms by history, we must actually measure orthostatic blood pressure and pulse to:

1. Determine whether orthostatic hypotension is really the cause of the symptoms.

2. Determine the severity of the orthostatic hypotension.

3. Determine if it is likely to be neurogenic (see below).

4. Monitor change over time with treatment.

The correct method

However, a correct method needs to be followed. Have the patient lie down for about 5 minutes. If there is no place for the person to lie down, then have the person sit and rest for 5 minutes. Then, measure the blood pressure and pulse rate. While measurement of the change in blood pressure from sitting to standing may miss some cases of orthostatic hypotension, it is still useful if the setting does not permit measurement of change in blood pressure from lying to standing (Shibao et al., 2013). So, if we can't do the measurement in the ideal way, we should still do what we can!

Next, deflate the blood pressure cuff but leave it on and have the patient stand up. Importantly, have the patient keep standing for one minute, measure the blood pressure and the pulse rate, and then measure again after the person has been standing for three minutes. Measurement at one minute evaluates immediate drop in blood pressure while measurement at three minutes evaluates a slightly delayed drop.

Standard definition of orthostatic hypotension

A drop in systolic blood pressure of 20 mmHg or more and/or a drop in diastolic blood pressure of 10 mmHg or more from lying to standing position occurring within 3 minutes has been the standard, accepted definition of orthostatic hypotension for many years.

A drop in systolic blood pressure of 20 mmHg or more has been shown to correlate with falls (Shibao et al., 2013).

Note: Orthostatic drops in diastolic blood pressure are commoner than orthostatic drops in systolic blood pressure. So, we should not forget to look at changes in both systolic and diastolic blood pressure.

When to measure

– It is important to realize that orthostatic blood pressure changes tend to vary at different times of the day and from day to day. So, if the orthostatic blood pressure is normal though suggestive symptoms are present, we should consider repeating the measurement of orthostatic blood pressure.

– We should especially try to measure it at the time of the day that dizziness or other symptoms tend to occur in this particular patient (Puisieux et al., 1999).

– Generally, orthostatic hypotension tends to be worse in the morning.

– If caused by a medication, the orthostatic hypotension may also be worst about 1.5 to 2 hours after taking the medication, when the serum level of the medication is at its highest.

– Orthostatic blood pressure changes are generally not related to meals but this may happen in persons with diabetic neuropathy.

What about 10 to 20 mm Hg?

It is not uncommon for patients with an orthostatic drop of between 10 and 20 mmHg to have clinical symptoms. Also, smaller drops in blood pressure of 10 to 19 mmHg predict greater drops at other times of the day (Weiss et al., 2004).

So, I recommend taking a drop in systolic blood pressure of more than 10 mm Hg seriously if a clinical picture suggestive of orthostatic hypotension is present. I myself have seen many such patients.

Change in pulse rate

Typically, the drop in the blood pressure is accompanied by an increase in the pulse rate as the heart tries to compensate for the drop in blood pressure. It is important that we not forget to also measure the change in pulse rate!

If the pulse rate does not increase to compensate for the drop in blood pressure, this usually suggests neurogenic orthostatic hypotension.

Management of orthostatic hypotension: Basic (level 1) strategies

1. Can the non-psychiatric medications that may be contributing to orthostatic hypotension be changed?

It is important not to be passive about non-psychiatric medications, just because we have not prescribed them. Ask the patient to discuss the issue with the other physician or, preferably, write to or call the other physician.

2. Minimize peak levels of the medication.

Since orthostatic hypotension is often related to the peak levels of the medication, minimizing the peak levels may help with this adverse effect. Change to a sustained-release preparation is highly advisable.

In addition, even if the medication does not otherwise need to be taken in multiple doses, to reduce orthostatic hypotension (and several other adverse effects), we should consider advising the patient to take the medication in multiple doses throughout the day.

3. Take measures to decrease venous pooling in the lower extremities

Explain to the patient the mechanism by which the orthostatic dizziness occurs to help the patient to understand and follow the recommendations for preventing and managing orthostatic hypotension.

– Avoid standing for a while without moving around

– While standing, cross one leg in front of the other–called the cocktail posture because many people stand like that at a cocktail party. □

– Intermittently tense the leg muscles to pump blood out of the veins of the lower extremities.

– When getting up, give the body time to adjust.

Patients should be warned not to jump up suddenly from a sitting or lying down position. Rather, they should rise up slowly while checking for dizziness. This is especially important in the first few days after starting a medication or changing to a higher dose. For example, a patient who has been lying down may sit up in bed, wait for a bit, then dangle her legs over the edge of the bed, then wait for a bit, then stand up slowly while holding on to something, then wait for a bit before walking. Systematic evaluation has shown that standing up slowly reduces the orthostatic drop in blood pressure (de Bruïne et al., 2016).

– If symptoms occur, try squatting if the person is able to squat. This may produce quick relief.

4. *Actively prevent dehydration.*

Patients should be told to drink plenty of fluids. However, there is no need to overdo this either. Patients can tell if they are drinking enough fluids by using these two methods:

a) They should prevent thirst rather than react to thirst. Thirst is the body's response to being dehydrated. If they feel thirsty, they are already dehydrated and need to be drinking more fluids to prevent this.

b) Check the color of their urine—it should not be yellow at all. If their urine is not clear like water, they should increase intake of fluids.

5. *Increase exercise.*

Two tips about what exercises to recommend:

a) Exercising in a swimming pool can be particularly helpful because the pressure of the water helps with venous return (Shibao et al., 2013).

b) Instead of exercises done standing up (e.g., walking on a treadmill), exercises done while sitting down may be preferred, at least initially, e.g., recumbent cycling, rowing.

6. *Drink 16 ounces of water.*

Drinking about 16 ounces of plain water in 3 to 4 minutes can reduce symptoms of orthostatic hypotension that occurs because a person has been standing for a while (Shannon et al., 2002). It is a "rescue measure" (Shibao et al., 2013). The blood pressure improves in 5 to 10 minutes and the benefit peaks in about 30 minutes.

The rapid benefit of drinking water is believed to be due to a sympathetic reflex due to the hypotonicity of the water (Jordan, 2005;

Jordan et al., 1999, 2000). Therefore, it should be plain water and NOT an electrolyte drink.

7. *Avoid falls!*

Patients should be told to not try to be "brave". I have often heard patients say, "I thought it will go away if I just keep walking." If a patient feels dizzy, rather than trying to brave her way through the dizziness, she should sit down or even lie down immediately in order to prevent falling. The dizziness should become better by sitting down. In cases of significant orthostatic hypotension, I tell patients that if necessary they should sit down on the ground rather than risk falling and injuring themselves.

Rescue measures

What if the patient is in a situation where they need to stand for a while (e.g., be at a party, go shopping). Are there things that can help right away? Here is a summary of some of them based on what was discussed above:

1. Drink two cups (16 oz) of cold water

It has to be water and NOT an electrolyte-rich solution. The cold, hypotonic fluid elicits a sympathetic reflex (Shannon et al., 2002; Shibao et al., 2013; Jordan, 2005). Orthostatic blood pressure improves soon and the benefit peaks in about 30 minutes after drinking the water. This trick can be helpful if the patient cannot avoid standing for a while.

2. Reduce venous pooling in the legs

– The patient should sit down whenever possible and, if possible, raise their legs

– They should keep moving around as much as possible. If needed and possible to do without embarrassment, they should slowly walk on the spot.

– Even without moving around, they can move the toes, tighten the thighs and buttocks, etc. Pumping the muscles increases venous return and reduces venous pooling in the legs.

– They should stand with the legs crossed (called the "cocktail posture" because it is similar to how people often stand at a cocktail party)

3. Bend at the waist

Doing this squeezes venous blood out of the abdominal (splanchnic) veins, so the patient should try to do this intermittently.

4. Squat down to the ground

Patients should do this immediately if they feel dizzy or faint This usually brings quick relief and can prevent a fall

What if these basic (level 1) strategies don't work or are not enough? We may have to move to intermediate (level 2) strategies.

Management of orthostatic hypotension: Intermediate (level 2) strategies

Based on a careful assessment of the risk-benefit ratio, psychopharmacologists are not uncommonly put in the difficult position of having to continue a psychiatric medication that is causing orthostatic hypotension. In such situations, in addition to the "basic" measures discussed above, other "intermediate" or "level 2" measures may be needed.

Abdominal binder

The cause of orthostatic hypotension due to psychiatric medications is that, on standing up, blood pools in the veins of the lower body. One way to reduce this is to compress the veins in some way.

When we think of venous compression, we typically think of venous compression of the legs. But, venous compression of the abdomen is even more effective (Subbaryan et al., 2019). The reason for this is that the capacity of the abdominal veins is larger than that of the veins in the leg. The blood supply to the abdominal organs (the "splanchnic circulation") is about 25% of the total blood volume.

Compression of the abdomen (alone or along with compression of the legs) has been shown to be more effective than compression of the legs (Smeenk et al., 2014). Compression of BOTH the legs and the abdomen was the most effective in improving symptoms of orthostatic hypotension (Smeenk et al., 2014). Yet, I find that mental health professionals don't know about or recommend this simple but effective strategy.

Compressing the abdomen by using an abdominal binder is easy. Such binders are not expensive. They are available in different waist sizes and in different heights (number of panels).

In the images below, we see the package the binder came in and the binder removed from the package.

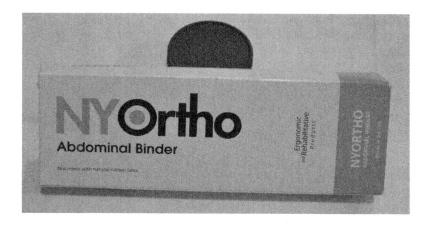

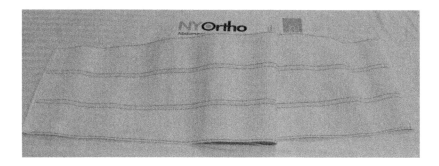

How to use an abdominal binder

Using an abdominal binder is a simple but effective way to manage orthostatic hypotension. But, it is important to follow the following tips in using an abdominal binder (Figueroa et al., 2010, 2015).

1. The patient must buy an abdominal binder of the correct size, based on the patient's waist circumference.

2. The abdominal binder must be adjustable. Typically, by using a velcro or hook fastener, the binder allows the patient to adjust how tightly the binder compresses the abdomen.

3. Compression of the lower abdomen (between the pubis and the umbilicus) is the most important.

4. Mild compression may be enough. Compressing the abdomen further may not be more helpful than mild compression (Figueroa et al., 2015) .

5. It must be worn BEFORE getting up from a lying position. This is very important to do if the abdominal binder is to be helpful.

6. It should be taken off before lying down. Otherwise, the blood pressure can become too high while the person is lying down at night.

7. Patients should be told that if dizziness occurs despite wearing an abdominal binder, they should NOT try to adjust the abdominal binder (Figueroa et al., 2015). That is unlikely to help in this situation. Instead, they should either sit/ lie down immediately or use methods of increasing venous return that involve tensing the leg muscles.

Compression stockings

These are not simply tight regular stockings but medical stockings originally designed to reduce the risk of thromboembolism. Therefore, they are called thrombo-embolic deterrent or T.E.D. stockings. The patient should make sure it says T.E.D. on the box. These can be bought on Amazon.com or at local pharmacies. See photo below.

Figueroa et al. (2010).

The T.E.D. stockings come in different lengths: knee (calf)-high and thigh-high are commonly available. The thigh-high and waist-high ones will be more effective but may be less acceptable to patients because they are hard to put on. Compression stockings also indicate how much pressure they apply; this should be at least 15- to 20- mmHg.

Custom-fitted compression stockings can also be made by prescription and are obtained at medical supply stores. These apply graded pressure, gradually squeezing blood from the lower leg upwards.

Although some studies have questioned the benefit of compression stockings for orthostatic hypotension, these studies were done in normal volunteers and I don't think we can necessarily extrapolate from them clinically symptomatic patients. The American Society of Hypertension recommends using compression stockings as one intervention for orthostatic hypotension (Shibao et al., 2013).

Increased salt intake?

Occasionally, if orthostatic hypotension is persistent and it is essential to continue the medication (e.g., clozapine), increased salt intake may be recommended.

Patients may be told to increase their salt intake with food provided that increased salt intake is not contraindicated for some reason (e.g., hypertension, heart failure, renal failure).

Alternatively, if needed, sodium chloride 1 to 2 gms with each meal can be recommended (Lanier et al., 2011; Kranzler and Cardoni, 1988).

Sodium chloride is available over-the-counter or online, most commonly as 1 gram tablets.

Note: If sodium supplementation is recommended, it is important to monitor not only the improvement in orthostatic hypotension but also for fluid retention. This can be done by looking for weight gain and for edema (Lanier et al., 2011).

[Optional to read: While not commonly done, a test is available to help decide whether sodium supplementation could be helpful—a 24-hour urine sodium level. If the 24-hour urine sodium is < 170 mmol per 24 hours, we may recommend sodium chloride tablets 1 to 2 g three times a day (Lanier et al., 2011). After one to two weeks, we can repeat the 24-hour urine sodium level. If sodium supplementation works, the urine sodium level should increase to between 150 and 200 mEq (Low and Singer, 2008).]

MYOCARDITIS

Clozapine-induced myocarditis or cardiomyopathy

Agranulocytosis is not the only medically serious potential adverse effect of clozapine. There are three other important ones. It can also cause intestinal ileus, seizures, and myocarditis. Mnemonic for the four: SIAM

It is absolutely essential that if we ever prescribe clozapine or see patients who are on clozapine, we should be aware of these three potentially very serious adverse effects.

Mental health professionals should be able to screen for it and identify myocarditis. We are not the ones who are going to manage it.

How common is it?

It is very difficult to know the true incidence because most cases go unreported and many cases even go undiagnosed. So, even though the reported incidence is between 0.02 to 0.2% (Merrill et al., 2014), the true incidence is probably more than that.

So, bottom-line— the true incidence is not known, it is thankfully uncommon, but still, it is probably more common than we think.

When is it more likely to occur?

An important thing to know is that the incidence is very different in the first two months of treatment compared to later on. The incidence between < 0.1 to as much as 1% in the first two months of treatment (Curto et al., 2016).

It then decreases to one-tenths of that during the rest of the first year of treatment.

So, 90% of the cases occur in the first two months of treatment (Citrome et al., 2016).

Is it dose-dependent?

No. It has been seen at low or usual doses as well (Citrome et al., 2016)

How serious is it?

The mortality of clozapine-induced myocarditis is about 25% (Curto et al., 2016), ranging from 10% to 50% (Citrome et al., 2016; Merrill et al., 2014).

If the myocarditis progresses to dilated cardiomyopathy, half of those patients die within 5 years of the diagnosis (Merrill et al., 2005).

What is the mechanism?

We don't know. It has been hypothesized to be a type 1 hypersensitivity reaction (Citrome et al., 2016).

When should we suspect it?

Early diagnosis is extremely important because of the seriousness of the problem and because delayed diagnosis has been associated with poorer prognosis.

Important! Often, the clinical features don't strongly suggest myocarditis (Merrill et al., 2014). So, we need to:

1. Have a low threshold for considering the possibility of myocarditis

2. Screen patients specifically for symptoms and signs suggestive of myocarditis. This should be done weekly for the first eight weeks.

Fever, palpitations, non-specific flu-like symptoms, chest pain, and shortness of breath occurring in a patient on clozapine should raise a strong suspicion of myocarditis.

Note: Benign fever (20% of patients) and tachycardia are common in persons who have recently started clozapine. So, to identify myocarditis, the presence of other symptoms should be looked for. But fever should not be assumed to be benign without evaluating the person for possible myocarditis (or agranulocytosis).

A narrow pulse pressure (systolic BP minus diastolic BP) of less than 40 mmHg and peripheral edema may suggest myocarditis.

3. Consider screening labs

What labs, if any, should be done to screen for myocarditis is not clear. Some have recommended checking serum troponin and C-reactive protein weekly for the first four weeks (Ronaldson et al., 2011), but this is not standard accepted practice.

What tests should be ordered initially?

If myocarditis is suspected due to the clinical symptoms discussed above:

1. An electrocardiogram (ECG) should be done. ST segment elevation may be seen.

2. Serum troponin (I or T) and Creatine kinase (CK-MB) levels should be done and may be increased, indicating damage to the myocardium

3. WBC count (for leucocytosis and eosinophilia) and C-reactive protein are also recommended.

If there are any abnormalities on the ECG or if troponin or CK-MB are elevated, the patient requires emergency evaluation by a cardiologist.

Which other tests may be helpful?

The cardiologist may consider the following tests.

Echocardiography: decreased ejection fraction, ventricular failure

Cardiac MRI

Treatment?

Clozapine should be stopped immediately.

The cardiologist would be the one to treat the condition.

Typically, they use beta-blockers, ACE inhibitors, and diuretics.

They may also consider using corticosteroids.

Rechallenge?

Most, but not all, patients develop myocarditis again if clozapine is restarted (Merrill et al., 2014). Yikes!

So, it is recommended that persons who develop clozapine-induced myocarditis should never be given clozapine again.

But we are aware that there are occasional reports of being able to put the person back on clozapine. If this is even considered, the patient should be referred to a tertiary medical center for this purpose. Very careful and specialized monitoring would be needed in such situations.

QT PROLONGATION AND OTHER ECG CHANGES

Antipsychotics and QT Prolongation

Second-generation ("Atypical") antipsychotics can prolong the QTc interval. Here is the ranking of four very commonly used ones from greatest to lowest propensity to prolong QTc.

Ziprasidone
Quetiapine
Risperidone
Olanzapine

So, contrary to popular belief, quetiapine is NOT very low in its tendency to prolong the QTc interval. It is less clear as to where exactly to place haloperidol in this ranking. One systematic study (Harrigan et al., 2004) put it above quetiapine, while a review by the FDA put it below olanzapine.

Antibiotics, Antipsychotics, and QT Prolongation

A colleague discussed with me a person who was being transferred from another hospital to ours. This person had psychosis, possibly schizophrenia. He had been admitted to the other hospital for a serious infection, which was much improved with antibiotic treatment that was continuing. We had to start him on an antipsychotic. What would you want to know before you decide on the antipsychotic and start it?

Well, I had a question to ask this colleague. I asked which antibiotic the patient was on. I was told that it was moxifloxacin (brand name Avelox in the US). Would you have any concerns?

Moxifloxacin so reliably causes QTc prolongation that the FDA uses it as the comparator when evaluating whether or not a new drug causes QTc prolongation!

In this medically ill person on moxifloxacin, I suggested that getting an ECG before starting the antipsychotic would be prudent. I also said that, if at all possible, antipsychotics with a higher risk of QTc prolongation should be avoided.

After this conversation, I discussed this patient with some other colleagues and realized that there was a need to review which antibiotics can cause clinically significant QTc prolongation.

If the person had done a drug interaction as I have been urging people to do, the risk of an interaction between quetiapine (which was being considered) and moxifloxacin would have popped right up.

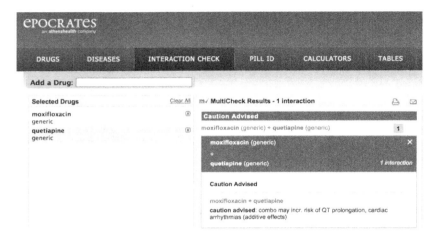

So, "Look it up!" is definitely the mantra to follow.

Even if we don't remember the list, we should also know there are some antibiotics that cause clinically significant QTc prolongation and require special caution when combined with an antipsychotic.

Which other antibiotics definitely cause QTc prolongation to the extent that they are associated with a risk of causing torsades de pointes? I mean not just hypothetically, but to a clinically important extent.

1. Macrolides: Azithromycin, clarithromycin, erythromycin

2. Fluoroquinolones: Ciprofloxacin, levofloxacin, moxifloxacin

3. Antifungals: Fluconazole, pentamidine

Some of these antibiotics are quite commonly used in our patients, so this drug interaction is important to remember.

SSRIs and QT Prolongation

In 2011, those of us who prescribe selective serotonin reuptake inhibitors (SSRIs), received some shocking news. The United States Food and Drug Administration (FDA) issued a Drug Safety Communication (FDA, 2011) stating that citalopram can cause dose-dependent QT interval prolongation. And then more news from the FDA related to this topic followed in 2012 and 2013. What did the FDA say and what exactly were the many things it said we should do? What about escitalopram? (Hint: you do need to be concerned.) What about other SSRIs? (Hint: there is one more SSRI for which the FDA has issued a similar warning.)

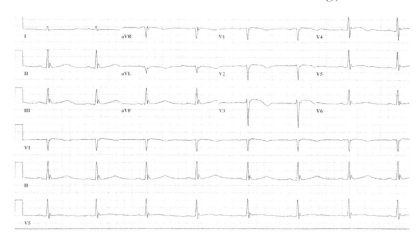

This 2011 guidance did not provide detailed recommendations. It said just that citalopram should not be prescribed:

a) at a dose > 40 mg/day, or

b) in persons with congenital long QT syndrome.

What was this based on? Two things:

1. The FDA said it had received post-marketing reports of QT interval prolongation and of torsades de pointes arrhythmias in persons prescribed citalopram.

2. It also reviewed two unpublished studies of QT prolongation with

citalopram and escitalopram. These were randomized, double-blind, placebo-controlled, crossover studies. Subjects in these studies received one of the following treatments: citalopram 20 mg/day, citalopram 60 mg/day, escitalopram 10 mg/day, escitalopram 30 mg/day, moxifloxacin 400 mg/day (known to produce QT prolongation), or placebo. These studies found that citalopram was associated with potentially clinically significant QT prolongation at 60 mg/day.

Detailed guidance about citalopram (Celexa®)

The next year, in 2012, the FDA (FDA, 2012) issued revised recommendations with guidance about different clinical situations. This is still valid as of publication of this book. The FDA's guidance about the use of citalopram can be organized under a few headings:

1. Patient selection

Citalopram is not recommended for patients who:

Have congenital long QT syndrome

Have bradycardia

Have hypokalemia or hypomagnesemia

Had a recent acute myocardial infarction, or uncompensated heart failure

Are taking other drugs that prolong the QT interval

2. Dosing

The maximum recommended dose of citalopram is 20 mg/day for patients:

> 60 years old

With hepatic impairment

Who are CYP 2C19 poor metabolizers (How are we supposed to know whether or not our patient is a CYP 2C19 poor metabolizer? The FDA does not say.)

Who are taking a CYP2C19 inhibitor

3. Patient education

Patients should be told to contact a healthcare professional immediately if they have symptoms like dizziness, palpitations, or syncope that may indicate a problem with the heart rate or rhythm

4. Monitoring of electrolytes and/or ECG

Serum potassium and magnesium at baseline and periodically in patients at risk for significant electrolyte disturbances

More frequent ECG monitoring in patients for whom citalopram use is not recommended, but is considered essential

5. Recommended actions

Hypokalemia and/or hypomagnesemia should be corrected before starting citalopram

If the QTc is persistently > 500 msec, citalopram should be discontinued

If symptoms like dizziness, palpitations, or syncope occur, further evaluation and monitoring should be done.

What about escitalopram (Lexapro®)?

In the studies reviewed by the FDA, escitalopram was not associated with QTc prolongation doses within its recommended range of 10 to 20 mg/day, so the recommendations for escitalopram were not modified by the FDA. However, I don't agree with the FDA's lack of concern about escitalopram. Why?

1. At 30 mg/day, escitalopram was associated with QTc prolongation similar to that with moxifloxacin.

2. If we look at data on persons who overdosed on escitalopram, the cardiac adverse effects are similar to those after overdose on citalopram (van Gorp et al., 2009). In persons who had overdosed on escitalopram, 11% had bradycardia and 14% had QT-heart rate combination considered to indicate risk of torsades de pointes.

We should note that the European Medicines Agency, the European equivalent of the FDA has made changes to the Summary of Product Characteristics not only for citalopram, but also for escitalopram. This agency recommended that the initial dose of escitalopram for persons > 64 years of age be 5 mg/day with the option to increase to 10 mg/day if needed.

What about SSRIs other than citalopram and escitalopram?

In 2013, the FDA also issued a safety warning for fluoxetine (FDA, 2013). It noted that it had received postmarketing reports of QT prolongation and ventricular arrhythmias (including torsades de pointes) in persons taking fluoxetine and recommended precautions similar to those for citalopram.

Can mirtazapine increase the risk of QT prolongation?

Vignette: A psychiatrist wrote mirtazapine for a cardiac patient on amiodarone. The pharmacist has objected because the interaction between the two can cause QTc prolongation (moderate risk). My EMR, Medscape, and Epocrates don't show this interaction. She quoted 'Micromedex.' Are you aware of this?

When evaluating the risk of adverse effects like QTc prolongation with two medications given together, there are two separate issues to consider–drug interaction and additive effects. Sometimes, additive effects don't show up in drug interaction searches.

So, in the situation faced in the above vignette, question no. 1 is whether there is a pharmacokinetic interaction between amiodarone and mirtazapine? And, question no. 2 is whether both these medications can cause QTc prolongation and so might have additive effects. The first question was addressed by doing an Epocrates search. How should we address the second question?

Any easy and reliable way to do this is to use crediblemeds.org. I recommend signing up for a free account to get the most out of this website.

First, I searched for amiodarone and got this result.

Crediblemeds.org uses risk categories for indicate how much the risk of

QTc prolongation and torsades de pointes is.

So, the red triangle icon indicates that amiodarone is known to prolong the QTc interval and is associated with a risk of torsades even when taken as recommended. The black hexagon icon indicates that amiodarone should be avoided in congenital long QT syndrome. In the first image above, a link is provided to PubMed articles about this.

But what about mirtazapine?

The yellow icon with a question mark indicates that mirtazapine can cause QT prolongation but is not known to cause torsades when taken as recommended.

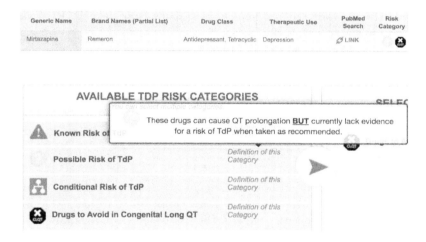

The Prescribing Information

The other place to look is in the Prescribing Information for mirtazapine. Here is what it says:

"The effect of REMERON (mirtazapine) on QTc interval was assessed in a clinical randomized trial with placebo and positive (moxifloxacin) controls involving 54 healthy volunteers using exposure response analysis. This trial showed a positive relationship between mirtazapine concentrations and prolongation of the QTc interval.

However, the degree of QT prolongation observed with both 45 mg (therapeutic) and 75 mg (supratherapeutic) doses of mirtazapine was not at a level generally considered to be clinically meaningful.

During the postmarketing use of mirtazapine, cases of QT prolongation, Torsades de Pointes, ventricular tachycardia, and sudden death, have been reported (see ADVERSE REACTIONS). The majority of reports occurred in association with overdose or in patients with other risk factors for QT prolongation, including concomitant use of QTc-prolonging medicines (see PRECAUTIONS, Drug Interactions and OVERDOSAGE sections).

Caution should be exercised when REMERON is prescribed in patients with known cardiovascular disease or family history of QT prolongation, and in concomitant use with other medicinal products thought to prolong the QTc interval."

The section on Drug Interactions in the mirtazapine Prescribing Information states:

"The risk of QT prolongation and/or ventricular arrhythmias (e.g., Torsades de Pointes) may be increased with concomitant use of medicines which prolong the QTc interval (e.g., some antipsychotics and antibiotics) and in case of mirtazapine overdose."

Bottom line

Above, we looked at how we might approach a case in which a pharmacist objected to the use of mirtazapine in a patient who is on amiodarone because this may increase the risk of QT prolongation.

Following the link in the crediblemeds.org search results to PubMed, we find the data suggesting that mirtazapine may cause QT prolongation are quite weak (Jasaik and Bostwick, 2014; also see Mago et al., 2014). But, the focus of this article was not to evaluate the truth of what is stated in the literature and in the Prescribing Information.

The purpose of this article was to how exactly to look up the risk of QT prolongation with any medication. I hope you were able to see how easy and quick it is to do this on crediblemeds.org? Please remember that website and use it whenever you need to check whether a medication is or is not associated with a risk of a) QT prolongation and b) ventricular arrhythmia. Also, crediblemeds.org lets us know whether this risk is present only under special circumstances or even when the medication is used as recommended.

The bottom line is that, even if this is rare, it is certainly possible that adding mirtazapine to amiodarone in this patient may put the patient at increased risk of QTc prolongation. In my opinion, if the FDA-approved Prescribing Information warns about a risk, it is advisable to take that warning into account. Also, the point here was that when given along with other medications that are known to cause QT prolongation, mirtazapine may increase the risk further.

In deciding what to do, we should also take into consideration whether the patient has any other risk factors for QT prolongation (e.g., age above 55 years, electrolyte imbalance, etc.?

Then, we ask: is mirtazapine really essential in this patient and worth the risk? Maybe it would be best to use a different antidepressant, one that has not been associated with an increased risk of QT prolongation.

But, if a decision was made in this patient who is on amiodarone that the potential benefits of prescribing mirtazapine outweigh the risk, this should be done in consultation with the patient's cardiologist. Also, an ECG should be done both before and after starting the mirtazapine and it may need to be repeated if the mirtazapine is increased to a full dose.

Does this drug cause QT prolongation and torsades?

On many occasions, I have needed to look up whether a particular drug is known to cause QTc prolongation or torsades de pointes ventricular arrhythmia. What would be an easy but authoritative way to do that?

For example, a patient of mine needed to be put on a proton pump inhibitor due to increased bleeding tendency with an SSRI, but reported that he had had drug-induced QTc prolongation on proton pump inhibitors in the past. So, I wanted to at least put him on an H2 blocker, perhaps famotidine (Pepcid®). How would I look up whether or not famotidine has been known to cause QTc prolongation?

The best source I know of is crediblemeds.org.

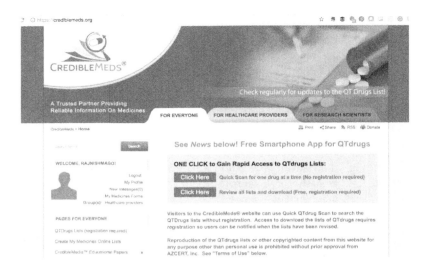

AZCERTor Arizona CERT, an independent non-profit organization, maintains the CredibleMeds® website and the QTdrugs lists of drugs that have a risk of QT prolongation and cardiac arrhythmias under a contract with the FDA's Safe Use Initiative to support the safe use of medications.

Free registration provides full access to the website.

For those like me who may have used previous versions of this database, Crediblemeds.org subsumes the previous websites torsades.org and QTdrugs.org. If you try to go to those websites, you will be automatically redirected to crediblemeds.org.

Clicking on "QTDrugs List" on the left side of the homepage brings us to the search page where we can look up any drug. The search results classify the drugs into those with known risk, possible risk, and conditional risk (i.e., risk only under certain circumstances). Possible risk means that the drug has been associated with QT prolongation, but currently lacks evidence of causing torsades de pointes arrhythmia if used as directed.

Note: if the search says drug not found, it means that the drug has not been associated with QT prolongation/ torsades.

So, I searched for famotidine:

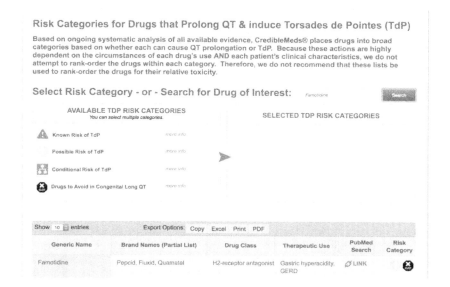

Risk Categories for Drugs that Prolong QT & induce Torsades de Pointes (TdP)

Based on ongoing systematic analysis of all available evidence, CredibleMeds® places drugs into broad categories based on whether each can cause QT prolongation or TdP. Because these actions are highly dependent on the circumstances of each drug's use AND each patient's clinical characteristics, we do not attempt to rank-order the drugs within each category. Therefore, we do not recommend that these lists be used to rank-order the drugs for their relative toxicity.

Select Risk Category - or - Search for Drug of Interest:

Famotidine   Search

AVAILABLE TDP RISK CATEGORIES		SELECTED TDP RISK CATEGORIES
You can select multiple categories.		
Known Risk of TdP	more info	
Possible Risk of TdP	more info	
Conditional Risk of TdP	more info	
Drugs to Avoid in Congenital Long QT	more info	

Show 10 entries   Export Options: Copy Excel Print PDF

Generic Name	Brand Names (Partial List)	Drug Class	Therapeutic Use	PubMed Search	Risk Category
Famotidine	Pepcid, Fluxid, Quamatel	H2-receptor antagonist	Gastric hyperacidity, GERD	LINK	

In view of the possible risk, we opted to use ranitidine instead, which was not found in this database.

Lithium's effects on the electrocardiogram (ECG, EKG)

A cardiologist colleague asked me a question informally about one of her patients. The patient has bipolar disorder was referred to the cardiologist by his psychiatrist because the patient was found, just by chance, to have a low heart rate. The psychiatrist told the patient that this may mean that he has some cardiac disease and asked him to see the cardiologist.

The cardiologist asked me, just to rule out the possibility, whether the patient's psychiatric medications can cause bradycardia, though the referring psychiatrist had not suggested that possibility. I asked what psychiatric medications the patient was on and she said lamotrigine and lithium. She also showed me the patient's ECG, which is shown in the image below. What do you think?

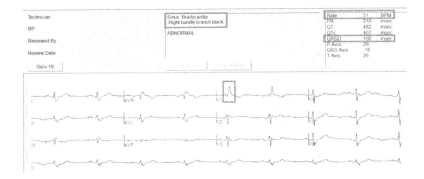

Various effects of lithium on the ECG have been described ranging from the benign and asymptomatic to the very serious. The effects of lithium on the electrical activity of the heart and on the ECG tend to be different depending on whether the serum lithium is in the usual therapeutic range or in the toxic range.

At THERAPEUTIC serum levels

The most common ECG changes with lithium at therapeutic serum levels are:

– T-wave depressions (flattening or inversion). This is the most common ECG finding associated with lithium treatment (Mehta and Vannozzi, 2007; Bucht et al., 1984).

– Sinus node dysfunction. This is the second most common ECG finding associated with lithium treatment (Mehta and Vannozzi, 2007). Since the sinus node of the heart is where the electrical impulse leading to cardiac contraction starts, this sinus node dysfunction is why lithium leads commonly to sinus bradycardia.

Some of the clinical characteristics of these ECG changes associated with therapeutic lithium levels are (Mehta and Vannozzi, 2007):

– Typically, asymptomatic

– Typically, not dangerous

– Typically, related to the duration of treatment with lithium and/or older age. Note that it is hard to tease these two apart because older patients have often been on lithium treatment for longer. One study found that nearly 60% of older adults who were on maintenance treatment with lithium had ECG abnormalities (Roose et al., 1979).

Are these changes present in the ECG above?

– We can look at the ECG report from the cardiologist to see if T wave inversion is present. But, for those who are interested, here's a simple explanation. In this ECG, we see that the T waves are inverted in aVR and V1. But, T waves are normally inverted in aVR (as seen in this ECG) and can be either upright or inverted in leads aVL, III, and V1. In all other leads, T waves are normally upright. So, the T wave inversion seen in this ECG—in leads aVR and V1—is not abnormal.

– Sinus bradycardia is, of course, present in this ECG. Bradycardia is usually defined as a heart rate of fewer than 60 beats per minute.

Based on everything I have noted above, at first, I said to the cardiologist that lithium is well-known to cause bradycardia even at normal serum lithium levels and by itself, this ECG is not a big deal. I like to talk in technical language, which is why I used the phrase "not a big deal." ☐

But, then, I looked at the ECG again and realized that there are other findings, which suggest we need to check a couple of things in this patient.

Other findings in this ECG

In looking at this patient's ECG again, we see a few other findings that have also been reported to be associated with lithium treatment. After reviewing these findings, I recommended to the cardiologist that the patient's serum lithium level and thyroid function should be checked. I'll explain why later. First, please look at the ECG image again and note that:

– The PR interval is slightly prolonged; it is 210 msec. The normal PR interval is between 120 and 200 msec (or 0.2 sec).

– The QRS complex is wider than normal. In this ECG, the QRS duration is 160 msec (see the upper right of the image). The normal duration of the QRS complex is about 80 to 120 msec.

– Right bundle branch block, is also present in this ECG.

– The cardiologist agreed with the automated reading that the corrected QT interval (QTc) in this patient was 467 msec. This is borderline prolonged.

Other ECG abnormalities associated with lithium

Other findings that may be present in patients being treated with lithium include (Mehta and Vannozzi, 2017):

– Sinoatrial blocks

– PR prolongation

– QT prolongation (We should note that though QTc prolongation has been reported in patients with a serum lithium level above the normal range, no cases of torsades de pointes due to lithium have been reported as of October 2019.)

– Ventricular arrhythmias.

Even more serious problems can be found in lithium toxicity including sick sinus syndrome and even cardiac arrest.

What to check for

I suggested to the patient's cardiologist that the patient's serum lithium level and thyroid function should be checked. Why?

1. Patients with serum lithium levels above the therapeutic range tend to have slower heart rates and longer PR and QT intervals (Hsu et al., 2005). QTc intervals of above 440 msec were found in 55% of patients with serum lithium levels of more than 1.2 mEq/L (Hsu et al., 2005).

2. Although this is not well proven, either way, at least one study found that sinus node dysfunction, which is present in this patient, is more likely with low thyroid hormone levels (Bucht et al., 2014). As you know, lithium-induced hypothyroidism is not rare.

Bottom line

It is hard to remember all the possible ECG abnormalities that may be associated with lithium treatment. We can look up the details if and when we need to.

But, here are SIX general principles that it is important for us to remember about lithium's effects on the ECG:

1. Lithium can cause MANY different ECG abnormalities.

2. The most common of these are T-wave depressions (flattening or inversion) and sinus node dysfunction (bradycardia).

3. There is a pattern in the possible ECG abnormalities associated with lithium that have been listed on this page—lithium can slow down cardiac conduction at every step—from the generation of the impulse in the sinus node onwards.

4. Lithium's effects on the heart can range from benign to very dangerous.

5. ECG changes can be present EVEN IF the serum lithium level is in the usual therapeutic range

6. But, ECG changes, especially the dangerous ones, are more likely when the lithium level is above the therapeutic range.

Clinical recommendations

1. There is no recommendation to routinely do ECGs in all patients on lithium unless some other risk factors are present. Neither the official Prescribing Information for lithium nor major Practice Guidelines recommend this.

– An international consensus practice guideline for bipolar disorder recommends a baseline ECG in patients older than 40 years of age or "if indicated" (Yatham et al., 2018). But, this recommendation is not linked to lithium or to any particular medication.

– The British Association of Psychopharmacology's guidelines for treating bipolar disorders (Goodwin et al., 2016) do not mention ECG at all.

– Royal Australian and New Zealand College of Psychiatrists clinical practice guidelines for mood disorders (Malhi et al., 2015) makes a general recommendation to do an ECG in patients with mood disorders because some psychotropic medications are associated with a risk of QTc prolongation but does not mention ECG with regard to lithium.

2. If an ECG is done in a patient on lithium for any reason and if some

of the ECG changes described in this article are found OR if bradycardia is noted, we recommend:

– Check the serum lithium level since it may be high, and

– Check thyroid function since it may be low.

3. There are two cardiac conditions that if a patient is known or even suspected to have, we should NOT prescribe lithium—congenital long QT syndrome or Brugada syndrome. These are both potentially very serious conditions and can even lead to sudden death.

When would we suspect that these conditions may be present even if the patient denies knowledge of having them?

– Unexplained syncope

– Family history of either of them

– Family history of sudden unexplained death before the age of 45 years

– Unexplained syncope or palpitations after starting lithium treatment.

[Optional to read: Crediblemeds.org (see image below) recommends avoiding lithium in patients with congenital Long QT syndrome.

Generic Name(s)	Lithium
Brand Names (Partial List)	Eskalith, Lithobid
Current TdP risk category	Drugs with possible TdP risk
	Drugs to be avoided by congenital Long QT
Main Therapeutic Use(s)	Bipolar disorder
Route(s) administered	oral, injection
Market Status	On US and non US Market
Info in Drug Label	
QT increase mentioned	No
TdP cases mentioned	No
ECG Recommendations	No ECG recommendation
Warning for use in patients with congenital LQTS	None

The Prescribing Information for lithium carbonate says the following about patients with Brugada syndrome:

"Lithium should be avoided in patients with Brugada Syndrome or those suspected of having Brugada Syndrome. Consultation with a cardiologist is recommended if: (1) treatment with lithium is under consideration for patients suspected of having Brugada Syndrome or patients who have risk factors for Brugada Syndrome, e.g., unexplained syncope, a family history of Brugada Syndrome, or a family history of sudden unexplained death before the age of 45 years, (2) patients who develop unexplained syncope or palpitations after starting lithium treatment."]

Hydroxyzine (Vistaril®, Atarax®) is associated with increased risk of QT prolongation

Anxiety and insomnia are present in a high proportion of our patients. Clinicians need and want more non-addicting options for the treatment of insomnia that we can use either alone or along with other medications. One such option has been hydroxyzine. In the past, I too have frequently used hydroxyzine in high doses for the treatment of anxiety. But in 2015 there was an important new warning regarding its use that completely changed how we should use hydroxyzine.

Hydroxyzine is a first-generation antihistamine medication. It also has anticholinergic properties.

Brand Names

Vistaril®, Atarax® (which has been discontinued)

Adverse effects

Common adverse effects include sedation, dry mouth, etc.

Warning!

In 2015, the European Medicines Agency, the European Union's equivalent of the US Food and Drug Administration announced that there is a small but definite risk for QT interval prolongation and torsades de pointes in persons taking hydroxyzine.

It recommended that:

1. The maximum daily dose should not exceed 100 mg /day in adults and 2 mg/kg/day children weighing up to 40 kg.

Note that this maximum dose is much less than the maximum of 400 mg/day approved by the FDA.

2. Use of hydroxyzine is not recommended for the elderly

3. If the use of hydroxyzine in the elderly cannot be avoided, the maximum daily dose should be 50 mg/day.

Some general precautions are also recommended:

1. Hydroxyzine should be prescribed at the lowest effective dose and for the shortest time possible.

2. Hydroxyzine should not be used by patients with known risk factors for cardiac arrhythmias or those who are taking other medications that may increase the risk of QT prolongation.

3. Care is also needed in patients taking medicines that slow the heart rate or decrease the level of potassium in the blood.

QT prolongation with hydroxyzine versus diphenhydramine

Question: Hydroxyzine has a QT prolongation warning in Europe. Diphenhydramine does not. Which [of these two] medications is more likely to prolong QT?

In thise section, I'll address the more specific question—How do hydroxyzine and diphenhydramine compare with each other in terms of the risk of QT prolongation?

Our discussion may also be of some value in understanding how we may look up and think about similar risks with other medications.

What does crediblemeds.org say?

I recommend crediblemeds.org as the best place to start when looking up the risk of QT prolongation with any medication.

In looking up hydroxyzine and diphenhydramine on crediblemeds.org (in August 2020), we find the following:

Generic Name	Brand Names (Partial List)	Drug Class	Therapeutic Use	PubMed Search	Risk Category
Diphenhydramine	Benadryl, Nytol, Unisom, Sominex, Dimedrol, Daedalon, Banophen	Antihistamine	Allergic rhinitis, insomnia	⊘ LINK	

Here's what the symbols in the right-most column mean: Crediblemeds symbols

 Conditional Risk of TdP

 Drugs to Avoid in Congenital Long QT

Here, TdP stands for torsades de pointes, a serious ventricular arrhythmia that is associated with QT prolongation.

So, crediblemeds.org is telling us that BOTH hydroxyzine and diphenhydramine are associated with a risk of not only QT prolongation but also, under certain conditions, of torsades de pointes.

But, it does not answer our question as to whether either hydroxyzine or diphenhydramine is associated with a greater risk of QT prolongation than the other.

What does the Physicians' Desk Reference (PDR) say?

For hydroxyzine, the official drug label in the PDR notes:

"Hydroxyzine is contraindicated in patients with a known history of QT prolongation, as post-marketing data indicate that it causes QT prolongation and Torsade de Pointes (TdP).

The majority of post-marketing reports for QT prolongation occurred in patients with other risk factors for QT prolongation/TdP…

Use hydroxyzine with caution in patients with conditions that may increase the risk of QT prolongation."

On the other hand, as of August 2020, according to the PDR, the drug label for diphenhydramine does NOT mention any risk of QT prolongation or torsades de pointes. Hmm. That's surprising, isn't it?

Possibly, this difference in the official FDA-approved drug labeling between the two medications may suggest that the risk of QT prolongation with diphenhydramine is less well established or less of a concern than with hydroxyzine.

What do published studies or case reports say?

Regarding hydroxyzine:

– The number of published cases of QT prolongation or torsades de pointes is much larger than with diphenhydramine.

– In the reported cases, patients either had at least one other risk factor for QT prolongation or had overdosed on hydroxyzine (Schilt et al., 2017).

Regarding diphenhydramine:

– The great majority of published cases of QT prolongation occurred with an overdose on diphenhydramine (or, occasionally, in the setting of significant heart disease). We should remember, though, that diphenhydramine is one of the commonest medications taken in overdose (Thakur et al., 2005).

Optional to read:

– Sype and Khan (2005)—QT prolongation after an overdose on 625 mg of diphenhydramine, no ventricular tachycardia.

– Thakur et al. (2005)—QT prolongation and wide-complex tachycardia after an overdose on diphenhydramine.

– Ramachandran and Sirop (2008)—QT prolongation after an overdose of diphenhydramine.

– Husain et al. (2010)—taking 3 g of diphenhydramine (that's 120 of the 25 mg pills) was associated with QT prolongation and non-sustained ventricular tachycardia.

– Shah et al. (2015)—50 mg of diphenhydramine was associated with QT prolongation but in the setting of very serious heart disease.

So, what's the bottom line?

– Unfortunately, as of August 2020, I could not find any study directly comparing the risk of QT prolongation with hydroxyzine and diphenhydramine.

– But the above review of various sources suggests that, to the best of our knowledge as of August 2020, the risk of QT prolongation or torsades de pointes with hydroxyzine appears to be much greater than the risk with diphenhydramine.

– For hydroxyzine, specific precautions have been recommended for managing the risk of QT prolongation.

– On the other hand, for diphenhydramine, in usual clinical care, no precautions related to QT prolongation have been recommended as of August 2020. Of course, if the patient has serious heart disease or another significant risk factor for QT prolongation, or if the patient overdoses on diphenhydramine, the risk of QT prolongation becomes clinically important.

RAYNAUD'S PHENOMENON

Question: How meaningful is the impact of stimulants on a patient with Raynaud's syndrome? An ADD patient of mine with significant Raynaud's was told by her internist to tell her psychiatrist (me) to please stop her Adderall [mixed amphetamine salts].

Can psychostimulant medications cause or worsen Raynaud's phenomenon?

Raynaud's disease versus Raynaud's phenomenon/ syndrome

Raynaud's phenomenon or syndrome involves temporary ischemia due to vasoconstriction, which leads to the fingers, toes, ears, and nose feeling cold and painful or numb after exposure to cold or stress.

When it is a primary problem, it is called Raynaud's disease (Belch et al., 2017) and when it is secondary to an autoimmune or systemic disease or to some substance, it's called Raynaud's phenomenon or syndrome. Raynaud's disease is the commoner of the two—80% or more of cases (Khouri et al., 2016).

Medication-induced Raynaud's syndrome

Many medications are known to cause Raynaud's phenomenon, the most common being beta-blockers (Khouri et al., 2016). Other medications associated with Raynaud's phenomenon include sympathomimetics (e.g., phentermine, psychostimulants) and clonidine.

Many cases have been published in which psychostimulant medications were associated with Raynaud's phenomenon (for example, Monteerarat and Pariwatcharakul, 2019; Gnavel, 2018; Bayram and Hergüner, 2015; Iglesias Otero et al., 2013; Syed and Moore, 2008) or blue toes (Al Aboud et al., 2011). The association between stimulant medications and Raynaud's phenomenon was also found in a case-control study (Goldman et al., 2008).

I have definitely seen cases of stimulant-induced Raynaud's phenomenon in my patients. And, colleagues with whom I discussed this topic also told me that they had seen patients in whom they had no doubt that the stimulant medication was the cause of Raynaud's syndrome.

But, it is believed that medication-induced Raynaud's phenomenon often goes undiagnosed due to clinicians not being aware that it is a possible side effect (Khouri et al., 2016). Well, that's not going to be us, right?

Clinical features of Raynaud's phenomenon

In Raynaud's phenomenon, after exposure to cold or emotional stress, there is a temporary ischemia due to vasoconstriction. This typically affects the fingers, toes, ears, or nose.

It is essential to the diagnosis of Raynaud's phenomenon that the affected part becomes pale ("blanching"; Belch et al., 2017) as shown in the image below:

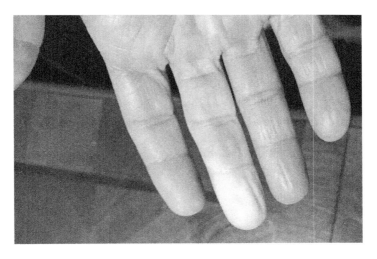

Blanching in Raynaud's

In many but not all patients, the classic triphasic color change—blanching leading to blueness (cyanosis) and then to redness—may be present (Belch et al., 2017). The affected part can feel cold, painful, or numb.

Other clinical features of Raynaud's phenomenon that may or may not be present are livedo reticularis (a mottled, purplish discoloration of the skin) and itching.

The image below shows marked cyanosis during acute Raynaud's phenomenon that occurred in a patient on methylphenidate after exposure to cold. Fortunately, after the feet were warmed, it subsided within a short period.

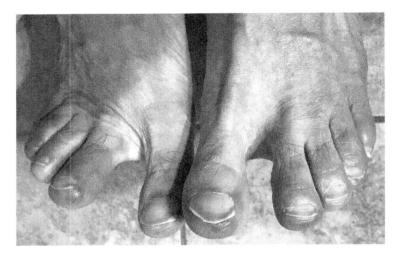

Stimulant-induced Raynaud's phenomenon and peripheral vascular disease

Here are a few things we can learn from the published literature about stimulant-induced Raynaud's phenomenon or peripheral vascular disease.

1. Though most of the published cases occurred in children and adolescents, these symptoms can definitely also occur in adults (e.g., Syed and Moore, 2008).

2. This can occur with both amphetamines and methylphenidate (e.g., Goldman et al., 2008; Syed and Moore, 2008).

3. Symptoms are more likely to occur within days or weeks after a dose increase, even in patients who have been on the stimulant for a long time (e.g., Syed and Moore, 2008).

4. While symptoms are typically mild, some patients may have severe or serious symptoms, e.g., tissue loss, gangrene (Tan et al., 2019).

5. Peripheral vascular symptoms, including Raynaud's phenomenon, associated with stimulants appear to be dose-related (e.g., Monteerarat and Pariwatcharakul, 2019; Bayram and Hergüner, 2015).

6. But, this does not mean that they occur only if particularly high doses are used. They often occur on doses similar to those used in usual clinical

practice.

Bottom line

There is no reasonable doubt that stimulant medications can be associated with Raynaud's syndrome and/or related peripheral vascular symptoms.

How common it is, I don't know. But, I suspect that it is more common than we think. I think patients with milder Raynaud's don't tell their clinicians about it.

Clinical recommendations

Immediate measures

– The patient should avoid exposure to cold by taking extra measures for keeping warm. For some patients, even a brief exposure to cold may be sufficient to precipiate an attack of Raynauds.

– Keeping the affected part warm is, of course, the most important thing. But, it is also helpful to keep the entire body warm.

– If Raynaud's does occur, warming the affected part is likely to help to improve the symptoms relatively quickly.

Stop the stimulant medication?

If the stimulant medication is stopped, the symptoms tend to improve quickly—within a few days—even in those who are positive for autoimmune antibodies (e.g., Syed and Moore, 2008). Note: It may take a few weeks for all the symptoms of peripheral vasculopathy to subside (Syed and Moore, 2008).

While it is easy to say that the medication should be stopped, stimulants are uniquely effective for the treatment of ADHD. Many patients are reluctant to stop the stimulant medication despite having Raynaud's or peripheral vascular disease as a side effect (Tan et al., 2019).

If the Raynaud's is occasional, mild, and easily prevented by staying warm, it may be possible to cautiously continue the stimulant medication. On the other hand, we must remember that if the Raynaud's is severe and/or frequent, or persistent vascular symptoms are present, there is a risk that ulcers and even gangrene may develop.

Whether or not the stimulant medication is stopped, the person should be referred to another clinician, preferably a rheumatologist, for evaluation and treatment. This may include the following steps as well as other evaluation and treatment.

Evaluation for possible autoimmune disease

While we don't know for sure, it is believed that patients who develop Raynaud's phenomenon and related symptoms on a stimulant medication may have some pre-existing vascular sensitivity that worsens due to the medication (Syed and Moore, 2008). In one case series, an underlying rheumatological disease was found in about 25% of patients, e.g., systemic sclerosis (Tan et al., 2019).

So, these patients should be referred to a rheumatologist for evaluation and for evaluation of autoimmune antibodies. They are often positive for one or more autoimmune antibodies, e.g., antinuclear antibodies, antihistone antibodies (Syed and Moore, 2008). Note: This evaluation should probably be done even if a decision has been taken to stop the stimulant medication.

Evaluation for other risk factors

We should also look for some other factors that MAY increase the risk of Raynaud's or peripheral vascular disease:

– Being on a vasoactive medication or beta-blocker

– Cardiovascular risk factors like diabetes, hypertension, or tobacco smoking.

If possible, stop or reduce any concomitant medication that may be contributing

If this is clinically possible, it may be helpful if the concomitant medications (e.g., beta-blockers, clonidine) that may be contributing to the Raynaud's or peripheral vascular disease can be stopped, or at least reduced in dose.

References: See https://simpleandpractical.com/side-effects-references

CHAPTER 4: DISCONTINUATION SYNDROMES

ANTIDEPRESSANT DISCONTINUATION (WITHDRAWAL)

Introduction

Antidepressant discontinuation (withdrawal) syndrome (ADS) is a relatively common and troublesome condition.

Antidepressant discontinuation (withdrawal) is not a newly recognized syndrome. It was first reported with imipramine soon after it was introduced (Haddad and Anderson, 2007).

Are antidepressants addictive?

I have had several patients who asked me if the antidepressant I was recommending was potentially addictive. Has this happened to you? If so, what did you say?

I have had several patients who asked me if the antidepressant I was recommending was potentially addictive. Has this happened to you? If so, what did you say?

Patients, their families, and critics of antidepressant medication often argue that the presence of troublesome symptoms upon abrupt discontinuation of antidepressants implies that they are addictive or produce dependence.

It is true that some patients have extraordinary difficulty getting off an antidepressant. And some patients have prolonged symptoms from stopping an antidepressant. These problems can reinforce the idea that antidepressants are addictive.

Also, when patients miss the antidepressant for a day or two for any reason and have discontinuation symptoms, they sometimes fear that they are becoming addicted to the medication and, therefore, decide to go off it.

At times, patients who experienced discontinuation symptoms with one antidepressant may refuse to take other antidepressants in the future.

Are these "discontinuation" symptoms or "withdrawal" symptoms?

The reason most authors use the term "discontinuation" is to avoid implying that antidepressants are addictive or cause dependence (Haddad and Anderson, 2007).

On the other hand, some people have argued that use of the term "discontinuation" is inappropriate because it minimizes the potential significance of symptoms that may result from stopping an antidepressant.

What we should say to patients and their families is that despite potential discontinuation symptoms, antidepressants are not "addictive." Why?

1. Patients don't take antidepressants to "get high".

2. There is an important difference between antidepressant discontinuation syndrome and withdrawal symptoms from other substances (Haddad and Anderson, 2007):

Once the discontinuation symptoms have resolved, there is no craving for antidepressants and patients don't feel a strong urge to return to taking the antidepressant.

Importance (Haddad and Anderson, 2007)

1. Suffering: these symptoms can range from mild to extremely bothersome.

2. Difficulty stopping the antidepressant

3. Non-adherence: When patients miss the antidepressant for a day or two for any reason and have discontinuation symptoms, they sometimes fear that they are becoming addicted to the medication and, therefore, decide to go off it.

4. Refusal of treatment: Patients who experienced discontinuation symptoms with one antidepressant may refuse to take other antidepressants in the future.

5. Inappropriate treatment of discontinuation symptoms if their nature is not correctly identified.

6. Misdiagnosis as adverse effects of the other antidepressant after switching to another antidepressant with a different mechanism of action (e.g., Haddad and Qureshi, 2000).

7. Misdiagnosis as recurrence of the underlying mental disorder.

8. Misdiagnosis as a non-psychiatric medical condition.

Risk factors

Antidepressant discontinuation (withdrawal) syndrome (ADS) can occur with all categories of antidepressants with serotonergic activity: SSRIs, SNRIs, MAOIs, mirtazapine.

Risk factors for ADS

1. Abrupt discontinuation of the antidepressant is the biggest risk factor for antidepressant discontinuation syndrome.

2. The other risk factor is antidepressants with a short half-life, e.g., paroxetine, venlafaxine. Fluoxetine, which has a long half-life, is less likely to cause ADS.

3. Persons who had ADS in the past should be considered to be at higher risk of developing ADS and stronger measures should be taken in these patients to prevent recurrence of ADS.

4. Persons who had adverse effects when the symptoms during the early phases of treatment with the antidepressant have been found to be more likely to suffer from ADS (Himei and Okamura, 2006).

Clinical features

Common symptoms of SSRI discontinuation (Haddad and Anderson, 2007)

1. Sensory symptoms

    - Paraesthesia

    - Numbness

    - Electric-shock-like sensations

    - Rushing noise 'in head'

    - Palinopsia (visual trails)

2. Disequilibrium

    - Light-headedness

    - Dizziness

    - Vertigo

3. General somatic symptoms

    - Lethargy

    - Headache

    - Tremor

    - Sweating

    - Anorexia

4. Mood symptoms

    - Irritability

    - Anxiety/agitation

- Low mood

- Tearfulness

5. Gastrointestinal symptoms

  - Nausea

  - Vomiting

  - Diarrhea

6. Sleep disturbance

  - Insomnia

  - Nightmares

  - Excessive dreaming

Management

Antidepressant discontinuation (withdrawal) syndrome (ADS) is a relatively common and troublesome condition. For mild symptoms, education and symptomatic treatment may be enough but for moderate/severe symptoms, it will be necessary to either restart the same antidepressant or switch to fluoxetine.

Educate the patient

Antidepressant discontinuation symptoms can really freak out the person. So, taking the time to explain what is going on is really important. Here are four points that we must make with our patients:

1. Tell the patient about what is causing the symptoms.

2. Important: Reassure the patient that the symptoms are not serious or harmful and tend to subside on their own in about one to two weeks in

most cases.

3. However, acknowledge that the discontinuation symptoms can sometimes take longer to subside. Tell the patient to call you if the symptoms persist or become more bothersome

4. Reassure the patient that the discontinuation symptoms do not indicate "addiction" or "dependence".

Symptomatic treatment if needed

We often assume that restarting the antidepressant is the only thing we can do or need to do. However, symptomatic treatment can also make the process of discontinuation less unpleasant for the person. Here are some options:

1. Benzodiazepine for anxiety

2. Hypnotic for insomnia

3. Ginger root one or two 550 mg capsules three times a day for nausea and vertigo (e.g., Schechter, 1998). These capsules are available in the US at GNC stores at low cost.

4. Ondansetron (Zofran®) 4 mg or 8 mg every 8 hours as needed for nausea, gastric upset, and headache (e.g., Raby, 1998)

5. Anticholinergic for gastrointestinal symptoms after stopping a TCA (e.g., Dilsaver et al., 1983)

Restarting an antidepressant

For moderate to severe symptoms, in addition to the measures listed above (educating the person about specific points and using symptomatic treatment), an antidepressant probably needs to be reinstated.

There are two main options:

1. Resume the same antidepressant.

This is the simplest option and works in most cases.

How soon will the person feel better?

The discontinuation symptoms are likely to resolve, or at least get markedly better, within 24 hours. In fact, this rapid improvement helps to confirm that the symptoms were due to antidepressant discontinuation (withdrawal) syndrome.

At what dose should the antidepressant be restarted?

The antidepressant should be restarted at the dose at which there were no discontinuation symptoms. For example, if a person was tapered from paroxetine 60 mg/day to 40 mg/day without a problem, but upon reducing to 20 mg/day, significant discontinuation symptoms occurred, we should increase back up to 40 mg/day. An increase to 60 mg/day, the original dose, is probably not needed.

Then what?

Once the discontinuation symptoms have stopped due to resuming the antidepressant, the taper can be tried again but this time at a much slower rate. In retrospect, if we had done a really slow taper in the first place, maybe we would have avoided ADS. But there is slow taper and there is really slow taper. We should always do a slow taper, but sometimes we need to do a really slow taper. See below for details of how to do a really slow taper.

2. Start fluoxetine instead of the original antidepressant

If the SSRI or SNRI is stopped and replaced with fluoxetine, this tends to suppress or eliminate the discontinuation symptoms that resulted from stopping the original antidepressant. Then, after several days or even several weeks, fluoxetine can be tapered off. The rationale for this strategy is that fluoxetine and its active metabolite, norfluoxetine, have long half-lives (about 5 days and about 2 weeks, respectively).

I think that in most cases we should initially we should resume the same antidepressant, then slowly reduce the dose, and then take a decision. If the really slow taper using the same antidepressant is going well, there may not be a need to add fluoxetine. But if the person is having problems, we should probably add fluoxetine. In general, I think clinicians currently underutilize the option to add fluoxetine.

How to do a really slow taper

The 10% rule

In difficult situations, it has been recommended that the medication be reduced by 10% at a time, but after every decrease, the next decrease should be 10% of the decreased dose, and NOT 10% of the original dose. The 10% rule can be hard to follow, except by using liquid preparations, but we can get as close to it as possible.

How exactly to do a really slow taper depends on the drug, the preparation, and the dose that the person is on right now. Here are a few options:

1. Some antidepressants are available as liquid preparations.

This allows precise measurement of the medication and very systematic reduction in the dose. Unfortunately, the antidepressants for which we would most love to have a liquid preparation (paroxetine, venlafaxine) are not available as liquid preparations in the US. *Note*: Paroxetine liquid has been discontinued by the manufacturer.

2. The half-life of the antidepressant is the biggest factor in determining how bad the discontinuation symptoms are. But, we can't change the half-life of the antidepressant, can we? Well, we can change the effective half-life by changing from an immediate-release tablet or capsule to an extended-release preparation.

Example: if a person is on paroxetine 60 mg/day, we can consider changing to a controlled-release preparation, e.g., paroxetine ER 25 mg two per day, bringing the dose down from 60 mg/day to 50 mg/day and changing to an ER preparation at the same time. Paroxetine ER is available in 12.5 mg, 25 mg, and 37.5 mg strengths.

Example: if a person is on venlafaxine 75 mg twice daily, we should consider changing to venlafaxine XR 150 mg one per day before starting a taper.

3. If the antidepressant is a tablet…

Gradually reduce the dose of the tablet by being aware of what strengths are available.

As an example, paroxetine is available in 10 mg, 20 mg, 30 mg, and 40 mg strengths. These tablets are scored and can be split to allow going down to half, or even quarter, of a 10 mg tablet.

When we get to the lowest tablet strength we can cut or even crush the tablet, as long as it is not an extended-release tablet. Then, a little bit of the powder can be discarded and the rest taken. Every few days, the amount of the medication discarded can be increased.

Crushing a tablet is not as good of an option as using a liquid. However, it may be OK for short-term use in certain circumstances.

<u>Pills that can be crushed</u>

If a tablet is scored, it is intended to be cut if needed. Such tablets are OK to crush.

<u>Pills that should NOT be crushed</u>

i.   We should not forget that many tablets are actually extended-release preparations. These should not be cut or crushed.

ii.   Enteric-coated preparations should generally not be crushed.

<u>How to crush a tablet</u>

i.   Use a pill crusher

ii.   Wrap the tablet in a clean piece of paper, fold, place on a hard surface, crush with a spoon or other hard object.

4. If the antidepressant is a capsule…

For reasons that we don't understand, some patients require an exceptionally slow rate of taper. In such situations, when down to the lowest available strength (e.g., venlafaxine XR 37.5 mg capsules) it may be necessary to open the capsule and ask the patient to take open the capsule, discard a little bit of the contents, then close the capsule and take it. Every few days, the amount of the medication discarded can be increased. Warning! Venlafaxine XR capsules can be opened in the manner but not all capsules can be opened.

How to add fluoxetine to manage ADS

As of publication of this book, there is no systematic study of adding fluoxetine to another antidepressant to treat antidepressant discontinuation (withdrawal) syndrome. Switching to fluoxetine was recommended as an option by a consensus panel on antidepressant discontinuation syndrome (Schatzberg et al., 2006), but no details were provided as to how exactly to do this. Based on my review of published case reports and on clinical experience, the following guidelines are suggested:

1. Do not add a full dose of fluoxetine to a high dose of another antidepressant.

This risks serotonin syndrome and, in some cases, a drug-drug interaction since fluoxetine is a potent inhibitor of several CYP450 isoenzymes.

There are three possible scenarios:

a) The dose of the other antidepressant is already at the lower end of the range and so fluoxetine can be added, e.g., venlafaxine 75 mg/day, duloxetine 30 mg/day, paroxetine 20 mg/day.

b) Or, we taper the other antidepressant down to bring it to the lower end of its range before adding fluoxetine.

c) Or, we add a low dose of fluoxetine and on the same day reduce the dose of the other antidepressant.

Here are examples of combinations that have been used safely in published case reports (Benazzi, 1998):

– Venlafaxine 75 mg/day plus fluoxetine 20 mg/day

– Sertraline 25 mg/day plus fluoxetine 5 mg/day

– Paroxetine 10 mg/day plus fluoxetine 2.5 mg/day

– Clomipramine 75 mg/day plus fluoxetine 20 mg/day

– Paroxetine 20 mg/day plus fluoxetine 20 mg/day

The way I think about it is that the total dose of antidepressant–fluoxetine plus the other antidepressant–should not be too high.

2. Let the person stabilize on the combination before starting to taper the other antidepressant. How long to do this for depends on whether it is clinically important to get the person off the previous antidepressant but it should be at least a few days.

3. If discontinuation symptoms are still present, increase the dose of fluoxetine.

4. After the person has been free of discontinuation symptoms for at least several days, slowly taper off the original antidepressant and leave the person on fluoxetine alone. The fact that the person is now also on fluoxetine is likely to make the taper of the original antidepressant uneventful.

5. Leave the person on fluoxetine alone for at least a week.

6. Then, either abruptly stop the fluoxetine or, if you want to be particularly cautious, reduce its dose once and then stop it. An elaborate taper is not needed with fluoxetine.

What are brain zaps?

Electric-shock-like sensations in the head have been described after discontinuation of antidepressants. These experiences are hard for patients to communicate clearly and they may describe these in different ways, e.g.,

– "Brain zaps"

– As if electrical discharges "popped" in the head (Campagne, 2005)

– "Brain shivers" (Cortes and Radhakrishnan, 2013)

– "Electrical-shock–like sensation in the brain"

– "Brain shocks" (Reeves et al., 2003)

– "Like a cattle-prod in my head" (Reeves et al., 2003)

– "Head shocks"

– "Electricity in the head" that "felt like the brain was shaking inside the skull" (Cortes and Radhakrishnan, 2013).

There can be several related symptoms

1. An electric-shock-like sensation. Often, the shock is perceived as occurring in or starting from the brain, but it can be described as occurring in the head. The electric-shock-like sensation is sometimes described as a "wave" spreading through the brain and even the body.

2. As shown by the term "brain shivers", a sensation that the brain is shaking or moving inside the skull can also occur.

3. Associated symptoms: There may be accompanying pain the head, dizziness or light-headedness, feeling disoriented (Reeves et al., 2003)

Factors that bring on the symptoms or make them worse

"Brain zaps" are related to abrupt or too rapid discontinuation of an antidepressant or to lowering its dose. In addition, even delaying taking a medication like venlafaxine for a few hours can lead to such symptoms (e.g., Campagne, 2005).

Some patients may say that moving the head or neck quickly (e.g., while getting up from a lying or sitting position; e.g., Reeves et al., 2003) makes the symptom worse. In that patient, the symptoms could be reproduced not only by active movement of the head and neck by the patient but also by passive movement of her head and neck by the examiner (Reeves et al., 2003). Others may report that moving the eyes quickly from side-to-side makes the symptoms worse.

Why would movement worsen a sensory phenomenon? Serotonergic neurons are distributed in relation to brain structures that control muscle movements and fire at the same time or in anticipation of gross movements (Reeves et al., 2003).

What causes "brain zaps"?

Presumably, "brain zaps" are sensory disturbances or paresthesias similar to those that can occur in other parts of the body. While it has been hypothesized that these are noradrenergic phenomena, they have been described in persons discontinuing either SNRIs or SSRIs.

Assessment

1. Asking the patients when the symptoms occur or are worse may help understand what is happening. If they are worse before taking the medication and better an hour or two after taking the medication, this would confirm that they are withdrawal symptoms.

2. The patients may be inadvertently taking less medication due to an error.

3. The patients may be delaying taking the medication and should be asked to take it on schedule.

4. A drug interaction may have occurred, lowering the levels of the medication.

Management

For a more detailed discussion of the management of antidepressant discontinuation syndrome, please see the previous section.

But, here are some brief tips.

1. Most importantly, if discontinuation of the antidepressant is indicated, the taper should be done even more slowly than usual because these patients may be more vulnerable to discontinuation symptoms than others.

2. We should make sure the person is taking an extended-release preparation since these are less likely to cause discontinuation symptoms.

3. An increase in the dose of the antidepressant is likely to improve the symptom of "brain zaps".

4. Another option is to give the medication in divided doses even if this is not otherwise needed, i.e., even if it is a once-a-day medication.

5. Atomoxetine 40 mg/day can be tried as a treatment and was reported to produce relief in the symptom within a few hours (Cortes and Radhakrishnan, 2013). Atomoxetine may specifically help brain zaps, though not with all discontinuation symptoms. It is not recommended as the first-line treatment for antidepressant discontinuation since most discontinuation symptoms are serotonergic. However, it could be considered when "brain zaps" are the main or particularly troublesome

symptom. After a few days, it can be tapered off.

DOPAMINE AGONIST WITHDRAWAL SYNDROME (DAWS)

By "dopamine agonist" we mean medications that are direct agonists are post-synaptic dopamine receptors. These include **pramipexole** (brand name Mirapex®), **ropinirole** (brand nam Requip®), **bromocriptine** (brand name Parlodel®), **rotigotine** (brand name Neupro®), and cabergoline (brand name Dostinex®).

[*Optional to read:* Rotigotine is only available as a patch and, as of April 2020, is only available as a brand name preparation ($705 per month).]

Some patients, when tapered off of a dopamine agonist, develop a withdrawal syndrome that is called, simply, dopamine agonist withdrawal syndrome or DAWS. There are several reasons why I think it is important for mental health clinicians to learn about DAWS:

1. Dopamine agonists are **used for the treatment of Parkinson's disease and restless legs syndrome**. Mental health clinicians do see patients with these illnesses because they often have comorbid psychiatric disorders.

2. Dopamine agonists are also used off-label (especially pramipexole) for the **treatment-resistant major depressive episodes in both bipolar disorder and major depressive disorder**. If we ourselves prescribe a dopamine agonist and then have to stop it, our patient may develop DAWS (as happened to one of my own patients).

3. In DAWS, the most prominent symptoms are psychiatric. So, it is **often misdiagnosed as a psychiatric disorder**. If we know about DAWS, we can help to correctly diagnose and manage this condition.

Clinical features

Symptoms and signs

The symptoms may be both mental and physical symptoms, but, mental (psychiatric) symptoms tend to be particularly prominent (Yu and

Fernandez, 2017).

The mental/ psychiatric symptoms may include **anxiety, panic attacks, dysphoria, depression, suicidal ideation, agitation, irritability, insomnia, craving for the medication, confusion**, etc, (Yu and Fernandez, 2017; Nierenberg, 2013).

The physical symptoms may include **insomnia, fatigue, autonomic symptoms (sweating, flushing, nausea, vomiting, orthostatic dizziness), generalized body pain, and restless legs** (Yu and Fernandez, 2017; Nirenberg, 2013). It is a bit odd but true that orthostatic hypotension can both be a side effect of dopamine agonists and occur during withdrawal from the medication (Nirenberg, 2013).

Case reports

Here are very brief summaries of two published cases of major depression developing after a dopamine agonist was stopped (Launois et al., 2013):

1. An 84-year-old man with no psychiatric history had restless legs syndrome (RLS) hat improved on pramipexole 0.7 mg/day. But, he developed impulse control disorder (e.g., teleshopping of antique books, sexual advances to his niece). So, the pramipexole was stopped and he was put on fentanyl for the RLS, which did work. Three weeks after the pramipexole was stopped, he began to feel very sad and apathetic, and had a loss of interest and pleasure. The depression did not respond to a trial of citalopram. When moclobemide was tried, it made the RLS worse. The major depression, unfortunately, continued for 10 months. Finally, he was started on rotigotine (another dopamine agonist) and the depression improved within five days.

2. A 64-year-old woman with a past history of depression was treated with ropinirole 3 mg/day for restless legs syndrome (RLS). Due to compulsive shopping and eating, the ropinirole was tapered off over three weeks and replaced with tramadol, which worked well for the RLS. But, three weeks later, the patient developed major depression, which was severe enough to require hospitalization. She had two antidepressant trials (fluoxetine and bupropion) but both of them worsened the RLS. She was then tried on a third antidepressant —agomelatine—but even 12 months later, she was still depressed. At this point, ECT was being considered but she was first given a trial of rotigotine. The depression went away within ten days.

These cases illustrate many points of interest to mental health clinicians:

– Stopping a dopamine agonist can lead to significant psychiatric symptoms

– These symptoms are frequently misdiagnosed as being due to a primary psychiatric disorder and treated with the usual medications.

– Antidepressants and anxiolytics typically do not work for the psychiatric symptoms resulting from stopping a dopamine agonist.

– But, restarting the same or another dopamine agonist typically results in the symptoms going away quickly.

How much suffering could have been prevented if the treating clinicians had known about dopamine agonist withdrawal!

Variable presentation

DAWS is extremely variable in many different ways:

1. It can appear **at any time during the taper process** (Yu and Fernandez, 2017).

2. The range of **severity of symptoms varies greatly** (Patel et al., 2017). In some patients, DAWS **can be quite disabling**, affecting the patient's ability to work, social interactions, family life, etc. (Nirenberg, 2013).

3. The **prognosis of DAWS is also very variable**. In about half of the patients with DAWS, the symptoms subside within days or weeks (Nirenberg, 2013). But, in others, the symptoms may last for months or even years (Nirenberg, 2013). In some patients (15% in one study, Pondal et al., 2013), due to the withdrawal symptoms, patients with DAWS may be unwilling or unable to stop the dopamine agonist medication (Nirenberg, 2013).

How common is it?

DAWS is believed to occur in **about 10 to 20% of patients with Parkinson's disease in whom a dopamine agonist medication is stopped** (Patel et al., 2017; Chaudhuri et al., 2015; Limotai et al., 2012).

DAWS has been reported mainly in patients with Parkinson's disease but **can also occur in patients with restless legs syndrome** (Shimo et al.,

2015; Launois et al., 2013; Dorfman and Nirenberg, 2013) or in patients who were on the dopamine agonist for off-label treatment of a psychiatric disorder. But, its incidence in these patients is not known.

Risk factors

Who are the patients in whom we should particularly look out for DAWS and be especially careful when stopping a dopamine agonist? Here are the risk factors for DAWS, listed here in no particular order.

1. The emergence of an **impulse-control behavior disorder** during treatment with the dopamine agonist (Limotai et al., 2012; Rabinak and Nirenberg, 2010).

Early on, it was thought that DAWS only occurred in patients who had developed an impulse-control behavior disorder attributed to the dopamine agonist, but this was based on only five patients (Rabinak and Nirenberg, 2010). This is still believed by many clinicians but is NOT true. But, still, impulse control behavior disorders are certainly a very important risk factor (Nirenberg, 2013). For example, in one study, of 84 patients who were withdrawn from a dopamine agonist, 13 developed DAWS (Pondal et al., 2013). In all 13 patients who developed DAWS, the reason for stopping the dopamine agonist was the development of an impulse control behavior disorder but this was true for only 41% of the patients who did not develop DAWS (Pondal et al., 2013).

2. A **higher dose** of the dopamine agonist at the time the dopamine agonist was tapered off (Rabinak and Nirenberg, 2010).

3. A **higher cumulative dose** (over time) of the dopamine agonist (Rabinak and Nirenberg, 2010).

4. **Parkinson's disease**. Though DAWS has also been reported in patients with restless legs syndrome, it appears to be much more likely to occur in patients with Parkinson's disease (Nirenberg, 2013).

But what is NOT a risk factor for DAWS is that it appears to be a class effect and is **not related to any particular dopamine agonist** (Nirenberg, 2013).

Diagnosis

It is likely that DAWS is greatly underdiagnosed (Patel et al., 2017). DAWS is also commonly misdiagnosed as indicating undertreatment of Parkinson's disease or is attributed to psychiatric illness (Rabinak and

Nirenberg, 2010).

Some key clinical features help to clinch the diagnosis:

1. The syndrome appears very soon after the dose of the dopamine agonist is reduced.

2. Other treatments (e.g., benzodiazepines, antidepressants) are not particularly helpful in reducing the symptoms.

3. Finally, what helps to confirm the diagnosis is that **if the patient is put back on the dopamine agonist**, the **symptoms of DAWS typically subside right away**.

Clinical recommendations

There is no specific recommendation for how dopamine agonists should be tapered (Yu and Fernandez, 2017) and no specific treatment for DAWS. So, what should we do?

– We need to **educate ourselves** about DAWS and **realize that it can be a very serious condition**. By reading this article, you have already done that.

Prevention

– Dopamine agonists should be used with caution in patients are high risk of developing impulse-control disorders (Nirenberg, 2013) or, in my opinion, who have a history of addictions.

– In patients who are treated with a dopamine agonist, high dose prolonged treatment should be avoided if possible since it seems to increase the risk of later developing DAWS (Nirenberg, 2013).

– Patients who are on a dopamine agonist, and a family member, should be regularly asked about possible impulse control behavior disorders. If such symptoms emerge, we should consider stopping the dopamine agonist because it is possible that doing this early on might reduce the risk of DAWS (Nirenberg, 2013), though this has not been shown in any study as of April 2020.

– When a dopamine agonist needs to be stopped, we should specifically identify whether or not the patient is someone who is at a higher risk of developing DAWS. The two main risk factors are: being on a higher dose of a dopamine agonist; having developed an impulse-control behavior disorder while on the dopamine agonist. In these **patients who are at**

higher risk, we should **taper the dopamine agonist even more slowly than in other patients—as slowly as possible—while carefully monitoring the patient**. This is the cautious thing to do even though the incidence of DAWS has not been shown to be clearly related to the rate of taper of the medication (Yu and Fernandez, 2017).

Treatment

– In case you think that maybe we can give **levodopa** while tapering the dopamine agonist, that may seem like a great idea but it **does not work**.

– If DAWS occurs, **going back to the previous dose of the dopamine agonist leads to the symptoms quickly going away**. Later, we can try again to taper the medication much more slowly than before.

– But, sometimes, we could be in the difficult position of having to continue the dopamine agonist *despite* ongoing impulse control problems. As noted above, in some patients (15% in one study, Pondal et al., 2013), due to the withdrawal symptoms, patients with DAWS may be unwilling or unable to stop the dopamine agonist medication (Nirenberg, 2013).

– We should realize that **no other medications (e.g., benzodiazepines, antidepressants, levodopa) are effective for the symptomatic treatment of DAWS**. The only thing that works is going back up on the dopamine agonist.

– Though I am not aware of any research supporting this, a Parkinson's disease expert suggested to me that we should consider switching the patient to an **extended-release preparation of the dopamine agonist**.

Why don't we give all patients the extended-release preparations in the first place? Due to cost. Here is a comparison of the prices of immediate-release and extended-release preparations of dopamine agonists (as of April 2020; source: goodrx.com).

Pramipexole 1.5 mg (30 tablets): immediate-release $9, extended-release $122

Ropinirole 2 mg (30 tablets): immediate-release $9.50, extended-release $25

– We should realize, and we should tell patients, that the **resolution of DAWS can take some time**. In one study in patients with Parkinson's disease, DAWS resolved in less than 6 months in 61% of patients but took more than a year in 23% of patients (Pondal et al., 2013).

References: See https://simpleandpractical.com/side-effects-references

CHAPTER 5: EARS

TINNITUS

Why tinnitus is important for mental health clinicians

Tinnitus is the perception of a sound (typically a ringing, buzzing, clicking, or hissing sound) in one or both ears without there being any external source of the sound. The sound may be perceived as coming from within the head or from outside the head (Tunkel et al., 2014). Patients often refer to it as a "ringing in the ears".

It is likely that you have had occasional tinnitus at some time? But, can you imagine how it would feel if the sound kept on going all day, every day? It would drive me nuts! Yet "chronic" tinnitus (that is, lasting for six months or more) is very common in the general population.

Why is tinnitus important for mental health clinicians?

1. Since tinnitus is a very common symptom, mental health patients report it, whether or not it is related to the mental health problem or its treatment. The simplest reason why mental health clinicians need to know a bit about tinnitus is that our patients sometimes complain of it and we need to decide how seriously we need to take this complaint. On many occasions, one of my patients complained of tinnitus and wasn't sure whether or not to refer to ENT. In the section below, I will share some tips about when tinnitus is more likely to indicate an underlying, possibly serious, condition.

Co-occurrence

2. Also, tinnitus is more common or at least more bothersome and disabling in persons with symptoms of anxiety, depression, insomnia, and somatoform disorders (Pinto et al., 2014; Belli et al., 2012). It has been recommended that all persons with tinnitus should be screened for psychiatric disorders (Ziai et al., 2017).

Note: A few persons with tinnitus may die by suicide. The reason for this is not clear but this is presumably due to the associated depression (Szibor et al., 2019; Jacobsen and McCaslin, 2001).

3. Tinnitus can be an associated symptom in migraine headaches, which, in turn, are often associated with various mental disorders.

Bidirectional relationship with antidepressant medications

4. As we will discuss below, some psychotropic medications can cause tinnitus as a side effect. For example, tinnitus is known to be a potential side effect of lithium. Also, tinnitus was reported in 1% more patients on desvenlafaxine than on placebo.

5. Tinnitus can also occur during antidepressant discontinuation (Clewes, 2012).

6. Paradoxically, antidepressant medications are also often used for the treatment of tinnitus (Belli et al., 2012).

Cognitive-behavior therapy as a treatment

7. Cognitive-behavior therapy is one of the treatments used for primary, persistent, and bothersome tinnitus (Tunkel et al., 2014).

Key things to ask about if a patient complains of tinnitus

When one of our patients complain of tinnitus, what should we do? There are some things that we, as mental health clinicians, should ask patients with tinnitus about because they will help us to decide two things:

– Does this person need to be referred for an audiological evaluation?

– Is it likely that the tinnitus is due to a serious underlying disease and the patient needs to be referred for a detailed evaluation, including imaging studies?

Before coming to things we should ask about, let us note that tinnitus can be (Tunkel et al., 2014a):

1. Primary: No cause other than possible sensorineural hearing loss can be found for the tinnitus

2. Secondary: The tinnitus is associated with a specific underlying cause other than sensorineural hearing loss.

Key things to ask about

A clinical practice guideline (Tunkel et al., 2014a) recommended that a "prompt and comprehensive" audiological evaluation should be done when tinnitus has any of the following characteristics, though we may recommend an audiological evaluation in other cases as well:

1. Unilateral

2. Persistent (has lasted for six months or more)

3. Is associated with hearing difficulty. Note: Persistent tinnitus is associated with hearing loss in the great majority of cases.

This does not mean that clinicians may not choose to get an audiological evaluation in other cases as well (Tunkel et al., 2014a).

Along with the three clinical features noted above, tinnitus is more likely to indicate a serious underlying disease when it is:

4. Accompanied by focal neurological symptoms like visual impairment, etc.

5. Pulsatile, that is, the person hears a thumping or "whooshing" sound along with the rhythm of the heartbeat. Pulsatile tinnitus may be coming from some kind of vascular disease near the ear, a tumor transmitting pulse from an artery to the ear, benign intracranial hypertension, etc. It is very important to not ignore pulsatile tinnitus because a serious, even life-threatening condition may be present (Sismanis et al., 2011).

6. Associated with asymmetric hearing loss (that is, more in one ear).

Important! Patients with tinnitus and the clinical characteristics discussed above should be referred for evaluation by ENT as soon as possible.

Optional to read: Tinnitus versus auditory hallucinations

Both tinnitus and auditory hallucinations are perceptions of sounds in the absence of a real external source of the sound. So, what's the difference between the two.

– Tinnitus is almost always a simple, stereotyped sound. By stereotyped, I mean that it is always the same.

– Tinnitus doesn't involve hearing voices

– In tinnitus, the person knows that the sound isn't really there. In a true auditory hallucination, the person is convinced that the sounds or voices are real.

– In tinnitus, the person doesn't interpret the sound in a delusional way.

Tinnitus associated with antidepressant medications

Our "go-to" source for looking up potential side effects

I think it is helpful to discuss how we should approach the question of whether and how often a particular symptom can a potential side effect of some medication.

I recommend that the first place to look is Simple and Practical's adverse effect handouts. These are available at the following link: https://simpleandpractical.com/aehandouts.

Why do I say that the information in the handouts we have prepared is particularly useful? Because we have carefully compared the incidence of a reported symptom that arose during treatment with a medication (called a "treatment-emergent adverse event") to the incidence of the symptom during treatment with a placebo. I take this "drug-placebo difference" to be an indicator of the percentage of patients in whom the symptom is attributable to the medication; that is, it is presumably a side effect of the medication.

Tinnitus as a side effect of bupropion?

When we look up the adverse effect handout for bupropion to address this question, we find that the drug-placebo difference for "ringing in the ears" during clinical trials of bupropion XL was 4%.

If we want more information about this, we can do a PubMed search of the MEDLINE database. When I did this, I found some published case reports of tinnitus associated with bupropion (Humma and Swims, 1999; Settle, 1991).

So, the clinical observation of tinnitus in persons on bupropion is spot on.

Tinnitus and antidepressants

There are four different issues to consider with regard to tinnitus and antidepressants

1. Tinnitus is known to be a potential side effect of pretty much all antidepressants, including SSRIs, SNRIs, TCAs, MAOIs, bupropion, and others (Robinson et al., 2007).

When tinnitus is a side effect of an antidepressant, if dose reduction doesn't work, it is at least reassuring to know that antidepressant-induced tinnitus typically resolves if the antidepressant is stopped.

2. Tinnitus can also occur during withdrawal from various antidepressants (Robinson et al., 2007).

3. When tinnitus is present in patients with significant depression (or anxiety), antidepressants may not only reduce the depression or anxiety but also the perceived severity of the tinnitus, though the data on this are not clear-cut (Baldo et al., 2012; Sullivan et al., 1993; Dobie et al., 1993; Sullivan et al., 1989).

4. But, should antidepressants be considered for the treatment of idiopathic tinnitus in persons who are NOT also significantly depressed or anxious? No, as of June 2020, there is no clear evidence to support the use of antidepressants to treat tinnitus in those who are not depressed or anxious (Robertson et al., 2005). It seems that antidepressants don't treat tinnitus as such. But, since persons who are depressed or anxious are affected by tinnitus to a greater extent, by reducing depression/ anxiety, antidepressants reduce the perceived severity of tinnitus.

References: See https://simpleandpractical.com/side-effects-references

CHAPTER 6: ELECTROLYTES

HYPONATREMIA

1. Which psychiatric medications can cause hyponatremia?

Oxcarbazepine, carbamazepine, and serotonergic antidepressants are the psychotropic medications most commonly associated with hyponatremia due syndrome of inappropriate antidiuretic hormone secretion (SIADH).

Several other medications may also be associated with hyponatremia at times, including other antiepileptics like valproate (Beers et al., 2010) and even lamotrigine (Lu and Wang, 2017).

2. What are risk factors that make hyponatremia more likely?

a) elderly, b) female, c) underweight, d) also on a diuretic, e) low baseline sodium (if known), f) had hyponatremia in the past

This is very important to know because hyponatremia rarely occurs in people without risk factors but is much more common than we may think in persons who are elderly and have these risk factors.

I like to say jokingly (but it is true) that "The risk is greater in persons with risk factors!"

3. When does hyponatremia occur?

It usually occurs early, e.g, within a few days of starting the medication.

4. What are early symptoms of hyponatremia?

The early symptoms are non-specific and can easily be missed. Check sodium if symptoms like fatigue, cognitive impairment, malaise, etc. appear. Very easy to miss if we not vigilant.

5. Diagnosis

Hyponatremia due to psychotropic medications occurs because there is excessive secretion of antidiuretic hormone (syndrome of inappropriate antidiuretic hormone or SIADH).

If hyponatremia occurs, we have to differentiate SIADH from psychogenic polydipsia. How can the mental health clinician do that? Easy! Check the plasma osmolality and urine osmolality at the same time. If the urine is concentrated but the plasma is dilute, it suggests SIADH. In polydipsia, urine will be dilute.

6. How should we manage hyponatremia?

The treatment of hyponatremia does NOT involve encouraging the patient to have more salt in his food or to drink rehydration drinks like Gatorade. We once had a patient with hyponatremia in our hospital who was started on intravenous normal saline by a medical resident on call at night! That is exactly the wrong thing to do.

Rather, the key to managing hyponatremia due to psychotropic medication (i.e., due to SIADH), is fluid restriction.

In addition, if the person is on a diuretic, we should change from the diuretic to a different antihypertensive if at all possible.

If the hyponatremia is severe or fails to improve with fluid restriction, the psychotropic medication that is causing the hyponatremia should be stopped.

7. What medication should we recommend after the hyponatremia resolves?

There is no clear guidance about this but here are the options:

1) If the same serotonin reuptake inhibitor is restarted after the hyponatremia resolves (i.e, rechallenge) the hyponatremia may or may not recur. If this is attempted, fluid restriction should be continued.

2) Similarly, upon switching to another serotonin reuptake inhibitor, hyponatremia may or may not recur.

3) If possible, the person should be switched to bupropion. While there are rare case reports of hyponatremia with bupropion, those patients were

on other medications that may cause hyponatremia. Therefore, I don't believe that bupropion can cause hyponatremia.

Another option is to start mirtazapine; it has a lower risk of causing hyponatremia than the serotonin reuptake inhibitors do.

How common is new-onset hyponatremia during antidepressant treatment?

The problem

Serum sodium is not being routinely measured after starting a serotonergic antidepressant in elderly patients. Also, the symptoms in persons with hyponatremia are typically non-specific and can easily be missed, e.g., fatigue, cognitive impairment, malaise, etc. This is why we must depend on systematic studies rather than clinical experience to answer the question: "What percentage of the elderly get hyponatremia with SSRI treatment?"

But, this is not an easy question to answer because it depends on the type of study, which population of patients we are talking about (different populations have very different risks of hyponatremia), how hyponatremia is defined, duration of follow up, and so on.

The range of reported incidence of new-onset hyponatremia during antidepressant treatment in different studies is so wide as to be ridiculous and meaningless. For example, one review concluded that the incidence of hyponatremia associated with SSRIs varies from 0.5% to 32% (Jacob and Spinler, 2006).

The proposed solution

I am using the term "new-onset hyponatremia during antidepressant treatment" because, obviously, we don't know that in every patient who develops hyponatremia soon after starting an antidepressant, the antidepressant was the cause of hyponatremia.

How can we provide some estimate of the incidence of new-onset hyponatremia during antidepressant treatment? I think we should focus on studies that:

– Are prospective rather than retrospective

– Are of at least some minimum size (say, at least 50 patients)

– Evaluate a well-defined population

– Measure the serum sodium level both before and after starting an antidepressant.

Do these criteria for deciding which studies to focus on for our purpose make sense to you?

Before you read on and see what I found based on these criteria, what would you guess the incidence of new-onset hyponatremia during antidepressant treatment is?

The findings

Above, fed up with the incredibly wide range of values given for the incidence of new-onset hyponatremia during antidepressant treatment, we decided to limit ourselves to certain types of studies. I was able to find only two studies that met those criteria. They are summarized in the table below.

Population	N	Antidepressant	Definition	%	Time	Risk factors
University-based outpatient research clinic[1]. Age: mean 75 (range 63 to 90)	75	Paroxetine, 12 weeks	Plasma sodium < 135 mEq/L	12%	Median 9 days (range: 1 to 14 days)	In the multivariate regression, lower body mass index and lower baseline plasma sodium level (<138 mEq/L)
Outpatient individual clinical practice[2]. Age ≥ 65 years	58	Venlafaxine, 3 to 5 days (with follow up of up of hyponatremia for up to 6 months)	Plasma sodium < 130 mEq/L	17%		

1. Fabian et al. (2004).   2. Roxanas et al. (2007)

So, that's our best estimate—in elderly patients, approximately 15% may develop low serum sodium levels after starting on an SSRI or an SNRI.

But, there are two other considerations:

1. What we don't know is—in how many of this 15 % of elderly patients is the hyponatremia severe, symptomatic, and persistent rather than milder, asymptomatic, and transient? It is probably a much smaller percentage.

2. On the other hand, the incidence is presumably high in patients at the highest risk:

– Elderly, especially females

– On a diuretic

– Low body weight

– History of hyponatremia in the past

Clinical recommendations

1. In elderly patients, after starting a serotonergic antidepressant we should monitor them for the first two weeks for non-specific symptoms that may suggest hyponatremia. These include fatigue, malaise, cognitive impairment, etc. If such symptoms are present, we should have a low threshold for checking the serum sodium.

2. In elderly patients at a particularly higher risk of developing hyponatremia on an antidepressant (as noted above), we should consider measuring the serum sodium (basic metabolic panel) before starting the antidepressant and about one week later.

How to diagnose SIADH

Several psychotropic medications can cause the syndrome of inappropriate anti-diuretic hormone secretion (SIADH). Most important among these are:

– Oxcarbazepine

– Carbamazepine

– Serotonergic antidepressants (SSRIs, SNRIs, MAOIs, TCAs)

Other psychotropic medications that may sometimes cause SIADH include lamotrigine, divalproex, and both first-generation and second-generation antipsychotics. Other than psychotropic medications, many non-psychotropic medications and many medical conditions can also cause SIADH.

SIADH presents with low serum sodium (hyponatremia) and non-specific clinical symptoms like fatigue, malaise, etc.

If a patient has hyponatremia, how should the diagnosis of SIADH be confirmed?

First, check if the person is dehydrated (dry mucous membranes, decreased skin turgor, tachycardia, orthostatic hypotension, etc.).

Next, make sure the person is not, the opposite, hypervolemic (edema, ascites).

Now, order these tests:

1. Serum creatinine--to rule out renal failure

2. Serum thyroid stimulating hormone (TSH)—to rule out severe hypothyroidism as a cause of low serum osmolality

2. Serum osmolality

3. Urine osmolality

4. Urinary sodium concentration

What will we find in a person with SIADH?

The person is retaining water so the serum osmolality will be low, typically less than 275 mOsml/Kg.

On the other hand, the urine will be unexpectedly concentrated. Urine osmolality will typically be more than 100 mOsm/Kg.

The urinary sodium concentration in SIADH is increased to more than 20 or 30 mmol/L while the patient is on normal salt and water intake (Verbalis et al., 2013).

What will we find in a person with polydipsia?

If the person is drinking excessive amounts of fluids, e.g., in psychogenic polydipsia, the urine will be dilute. That is, urine osmolality will also be low—less than 100 mOsm/Kg—and the urinary sodium concentration will also be low—less than 20 mmol/L.

METABOLIC ACIDOSIS

Introduction

You have probably read or heard at some time or the other that some medications used by mental health clinicians (on- or off-label) can cause "metabolic acidosis."

Which psychotropics medications can cause metabolic acidosis?

1. Topiramate is the most important one of these in the sense that metabolic acidosis, even if mild and asymptomatic, is more common with topiramate and is rare with the other medications discussed below.

2. Second-generation antipsychotics

Several case reports have been published of diabetic ketoacidosis (a form of metabolic acidosis) caused by antipsychotic medications.

3. Metformin

Metformin is often used off-label by mental health clinicians for the treatment of antipsychotic-induced weight gain. In rare cases, it can cause lactic acidosis, which is a form of metabolic acidosis.

4. Lithium has also been reported to cause metabolic acidosis in rare cases due to its effects on the kidney (specifically, renal tubular acidosis).

What does metabolic acidosis mean? As opposed to what other type of acidosis?

We read that topiramate causes "normal anion gap" metabolic acidosis. What does the "normal anion gap" mean and how would we know?

We need to understand at least the basic concepts so that we can identify normal anion gap metabolic acidosis when we see it in our patients' lab results.

What is "acidosis"?

Very briefly, let us remind ourselves that:

– The pH of the blood (approximately 7.4) needs to be maintained very precisely—within the range of 7.35 to 7.45. The body has many ways of doing that, including breathing and kidney function. When the blood is more acidic than normal, we call it "acidosis."

– Carbon dioxide (CO_2) is central to acid-base balance in the body because it can combine with water (H_2O) to make carbonic acid (H_2CO_3), which can then dissociate into hydrogen ions ($H+$) and bicarbonate ions (HCO_3-). Hydrogen ions are, of course, what make something acidic. And, bicarbonate ions can counteract the acidity if they combine with hydrogen ions and form carbonic acid that dissociates into CO_2 and water. Topiramate inhibits the enzyme carbonic anhydrase that catalyzes the conversion of carbon dioxide plus water into hydrogen and bicarbonate ions. That conversion is necessary to allow the kidneys to excrete hydrogen ions while reabsorbing the bicarbonate ions. So, serum bicarbonate levels decrease. We can easily see this because the basic metabolic panel laboratory test (sometimes called the "Chem 7") shows the bicarbonate level in the form of total carbon dioxide. Notice that in the basic metabolic panel result from any of your patients.

– Acidosis can occur if breathing is impaired and too much CO_2 is being retained in the body, in which case we say that it is "respiratory acidosis." Or, it can occur if there is an increase in acid (too much being produced or too little being excreted) OR if there is too little bicarbonate (too much being excreted by the kidneys or too little being produced by the kidneys), in which case we call it "metabolic acidosis."

Having refreshed our memories about this extremely brief summary of what acidosis is, we are ready to move on to the next step in our understanding. Next, please read the section below:

What is the anion gap and how can we easily calculate it from the lab results?

After reading that, you will be able to come back and understand the next section (below).

Two types of metabolic acidosis

Metabolic acidosis can be of two types (Sinha et al., 2018): High anion gap metabolic acidosis and normal anion gap metabolic acidosis. The reason this is important is that the anion gap is easy to calculate and the causes of the two type of metabolic acidosis are different. For example, topiramate causes normal anion gap metabolic acidosis. So, if the anion gap is high, that should alert us that we need to look for a different cause.

1. High anion gap metabolic acidosis

This is also called increased anion gap metabolic acidosis. It is caused by increased acid due to:

– Increased production of acid in the body (e.g., ketoacidosis due to diabetes, alcohol abuse, starvation, etc.; lactic acidosis, which may be caused by metformin in rare cases)

– Taking an acidic substance in toxic amounts, or

– A decrease in excretion of acid by the kidney (kidney disease).

2. Normal anion gap metabolic acidosis

This is caused by the increased loss of bicarbonate from the body, either through the kidney (kidney disease, diuretics, carbonic anhydrase inhibitors like topiramate and acetazolamide) or from the gastrointestinal tract (e.g., severe diarrhea, laxative abuse).

Important! There are several other possible causes of high anion gap or normal anion gap metabolic acidosis and I have given only a few examples of them.

Optional to read

Causes of high or increased anion gap metabolic acidosis include (Centor, 1990):

– Lactic acidosis

– Ketoacidosis, including diabetic

– Renal failure

– Toxins: Alcohol, methanol, ethylene glycol, paraldehyde, salicylates]

Causes of normal anion gap metabolic acidosis include (Centor, 1990):

Diarrhea

Acetazolamide

Urinary tract—bowel connections

Ileal conduit

Renal tubular acidosis □ □

Dilutional acidosis

Intake of acid (including hyperalimentation)

How to monitor for possible metabolic acidosis

You have probably read or heard at some time or the other that some medications used by mental health clinicians (on- or off-label) can cause "metabolic acidosis." Topiramate is probably the most important one of these.

Some standard textbooks recommend monitoring for clinical symptoms of metabolic acidosis and, if they occur, reducing the dose of topiramate or stopping it. But, I cannot agree with this on two counts:

1. *Monitoring*: We need to monitor for topiramate-induced metabolic acidosis not only by asking about possible clinical symptoms that may be present in metabolic acidosis but also by periodically checking the serum bicarbonate level in all patients who are on topiramate.

The Prescribing Information for topiramate (brand name Topamax), which is sometimes prescribed off-label by mental health clinicians, carries a warning:

"Metabolic acidosis: baseline and periodic measurement of serum bicarbonate is recommended; consider dose reduction or discontinuation of TOPAMAX if clinically appropriate."

Notice that the Prescribing Information, a legally very important document, states pretty clearly that the lab monitoring should be done.

Unfortunately, many mental health clinicians who have patients on topiramate may not be keeping an eye on serum bicarbonate levels and identifying mild, asymptomatic metabolic acidosis caused by topiramate. That brings me to my second disagreement with what some standard textbooks recommend.

2. *When is metabolic acidosis due to topiramate clinically significant?* Even mild, asymptomatic metabolic acidosis due to topiramate matters because the changes in urine pH and chemistry can lead to the formation of kidney stones in as many as 1 to 2% of patients. That's a serious matter, isn't it?

This is why we should regularly monitor the serum bicarbonate level in all patients who are on topiramate. But how?

How to monitor serum bicarbonate

I used to wonder how we should test for the serum bicarbonate level until I realized that it had always been right before my eyes.

One of the items in the test panels called Basic Metabolic Panel (BMP; sometimes also called the Chem 7) and the Comprehensive Metabolic Panel (a combination of the BMP and hepatic function tests), is the "Carbon dioxide" level, also called the "Carbon dioxide, Total."

For example, see the lab test result below:

Component	Value	Ref Range
SODIUM	133	136 - 145 mmol/L
POTASSIUM	3.8	3.5 - 5.1 mmol/L
CHLORIDE	97	98 - 107 mmol/L
CARBON DIOXIDE	25	21 - 31 mmol/L
BUN	6	7 - 18 mg/dL
CREATININE	0.78	0.5 - 1.1 mg/dL
GLUCOSE	70	74 - 100 mg/dL

But, you must be thinking, we want the serum bicarbonate level and this is the (total) carbon dioxide level. How are they related? Answer: The total carbon dioxide is used as a very good estimate of the serum bicarbonate level. Let me explain why.

We know that carbon dioxide (CO_2) combines with water (H_2O) to make carbonic acid (H2CO3), which can then dissociate into hydrogen ions (H^+) and bicarbonate ions ($HCO3^-$). The total carbon dioxide level that we see in the lab test results includes (Centor, 1990):

1. Serum bicarbonate

2. Carbonic acid

3. Carbon dioxide (dissolved in the blood).

About 95% of this total carbon dioxide is the serum bicarbonate (Centor, 1990). That is why the total carbon dioxide is a good estimate of the serum bicarbonate level.

Important! While drug-induced acidosis, a form of metabolic acidosis, is identified by a low bicarbonate level, in a medically ill patient, an arterial blood gas sample needs to be obtained so that pH and blood gases can be measured for a complete evaluation of acid-base balance. This is because the acid-base balance also depends on respiration. A low carbon dioxide level can be due to metabolic acidosis but can also occur as compensation for a respiratory problem. But, in mental health outpatients who do not have any acute general medical illness, we generally assume that the low carbon dioxide is due to metabolic acidosis.

If low bicarbonate is found on the basic metabolic panel (or comprehensive metabolic panel), the next step is to calculate the anion gap, which helps to suggest the possible reason for the low bicarbonate.

What is the anion gap and how can we easily calculate it from the lab results

We noted above that measuring total carbon dioxide level, which is included in the Basic Metabolic Panel and the Comprehensive Metabolic Panel, is a very good estimate of serum bicarbonate. And, that in the absence of respiratory problems, a low serum bicarbonate level generally indicates metabolic acidosis.

If a low total carbon dioxide level is found, the immediate next step is to calculate the anion gap because whether the anion gap is high or normal suggests what the cause of the metabolic acidosis might be.

But, let me back up and explain what the anion gap is and how we calculate it.

What is the anion gap?

In the basic metabolic panel result, the positively charged ion that is present in the highest concentration is sodium. For example, the potassium concentration is much lower by comparison. The sodium concentration is approximately 140 mmol/L while the potassium concentration is only approximately 4 mmol/L.

The negatively charged ions that are present in the highest concentration are chloride and bicarbonate (represented as total carbon dioxide).

Obviously, the positive and negative charges on ions in the blood have to be equal to maintain blood as electrochemically neutral. But, when we look at a patient's laboratory results, we are not looking at ALL positively and negatively charged ions. That is why though, in the body, the anions (negatively charged ions) and cations (positively charged ions) cancel each other out, when looking at the patient's laboratory result, there appears to be an "anion gap."

What I mean is that when we look at the lab result and add together the concentrations of chloride and CO_2 (the main two negatively charged ions), the total is less than the sodium concentration. That difference is called the anion gap. It is present because there are other negatively charged ions that we are not measuring. But, the important point is that there is a normal range for the anion gap. Normally, the anion gap is about 3 to 12. Whether the anion gap is normal or increased is an important indicator of what the cause of the metabolic acidosis might be.

Calculating the anion gap

Most laboratories (e.g., LabCorp) do not provide the calculated anion gap along with the results of the Basic Metabolic Panel and the Comprehensive Metabolic Panel. But, calculating the anion gap is extremely easy once we know how.

We just add the chloride plus the CO_2. Then subtract that sum from the sodium. That is—Sodium minus (chloride plus CO_2). This gives us the anion gap because sodium is the main positively charged ion and the main negatively charged ions are chloride and bicarbonate (which is estimated by measuring the total carbon dioxide).

Occasionally, the laboratory result gives us the calculated anion gap as in the results below, which are from one of my own patients:

Component	Your Value	Standard Range
Glucose	Your Value 158 mg/dL	Standard Range 70 - 99 mg/dL
Urea Nitrogen	Your Value 11 mg/dL	Standard Range 8 - 20 mg/dL
Creatinine	Your Value 0.53 mg/dL	Standard Range 0.44 - 1.03 mg/dL
Sodium	Your Value 130 mmol/L	Standard Range 136 - 144 mmol/L
Potassium	Your Value 4.6 mmol/L	Standard Range 3.6 - 5.1 mmol/L
Chloride	Your Value 95 mmol/L	Standard Range 101 - 111 mmol/L
Carbon Dioxide	Your Value 27 mmol/L	Standard Range 22 - 32 mmol/L
Anion Gap	Your Value 8	Standard Range 3 - 12

Of course, we could have easily calculated the anion gap ourselves. From the test result above, we add the chloride (95) plus the carbon dioxide (27), which comes to 122. We then subtract this 122 from the sodium concentration (130) to get the anion gap, which is 8. Easy-peasy!

Tips on using the anion gap

We noted above that the normal anion gap is about 3 to 12 mmol/L. But, here are some more clinically-important points about what the normal anion gap is:

– For a particular individual, we can consider the anion gap from that

Side Effects of Psychiatric Medications

person's baseline labs (before going on the medication that may be causing metabolic acidosis) as being the "normal" anion gap for that person.

– Among the anions that we are not considering in calculating the anion gap, albumin is one of the most important ones. So, if serum albumin is low, we have to correct for that in determining the anion gap. We use this simple formula [2.5 X (4 – albumin)] and add that number to the anion gap we had calculated in the usual way.

– For the purposes of using the anion gap (normal versus high) to identify the possible causes of the metabolic acidosis, we can consider an anion gap of 20 mmol/L or more to be "high".

Two types of metabolic acidosis

Now, coming to why mental health clinicians are bothering to learn about the anion gap. Metabolic acidosis can be of two types (Sinha et al., 2018): High anion gap metabolic acidosis and normal anion gap metabolic acidosis. The reason this is important is that the causes of the two type of metabolic acidosis are different.

For example, topiramate causes normal anion gap metabolic acidosis. So, if, in a patient on topiramate, the anion gap is high instead of normal, that should alert us that we need to look for a cause other than topiramate. Instead of the metabolic acidosis being due to topiramate, the patient could have a serious illness that is causing the high anion gap metabolic acidosis.

Once we have looked at the anion gap and identified that the person may have either high anion gap metabolic acidosis or normal anion gap metabolic acidosis, we must refer the person for treatment elsewhere. The rest is not for mental health clinicians to evaluate or treat. So, let's end our discussion of anion gap by looking at an example of each type of metabolic acidosis and some examples of possible causes of each type.

High anion gap metabolic acidosis

This is also called increased anion gap metabolic acidosis. Here's an example:

```
Comp. Metabolic Panel (14)
Glucose                      89              mg/dL         65 -  99
BUN                          11              mg/dL          6 -  20
Creatinine                 0.99              mg/dL       0.76 - 1.27
eGFR If NonAfricn Am        109         mL/min/1.73              >59
eGFR If Africn Am           126         mL/min/1.73              >59
BUN/Creatinine Ratio         11                            9 -  20
Sodium                      138             mmol/L        134 - 144
Potassium                   4.0             mmol/L        3.5 - 5.2
Chloride                    101             mmol/L         96 - 106
Carbon Dioxide, Total        17      Low    mmol/L         20 -  29
Calcium                     8.8              mg/dL        8.7 - 10.2
Protein, Total              6.6               g/dL        6.0 - 8.5
Albumin                     4.2               g/dL        3.5 - 5.5
Globulin, Total             2.4               g/dL        1.5 - 4.5
A/G Ratio                   1.8                           1.2 - 2.2
Bilirubin, Total            0.4              mg/dL        0.0 - 1.2
Alkaline Phosphatase        108               IU/L         39 - 117
AST (SGOT)                   62      High      IU/L          0 -  40
ALT (SGPT)                   72      High      IU/L          0 -  44
```

High anion gap metabolic acidosis is caused by increased acid. Examples of possible causes include:

– Increased production of acid in the body (e.g., ketoacidosis due to diabetes, alcohol abuse, starvation, etc.; lactic acidosis, which may be caused by metformin in rare cases)

– Taking an acidic substance in toxic amounts, or

– A decrease in excretion of acid by the kidney (kidney disease).

Normal anion gap metabolic acidosis

Here's an example:

TESTS	RESULT	FLAG	UNITS	REFERENCE INTERVAL
Basic Metabolic Panel (8)				
Glucose	111	High	mg/dL	65 - 99
BUN	8		mg/dL	6 - 20
Creatinine	0.87		mg/dL	0.57 - 1.00
eGFR If NonAfricn Am	92		mL/min/1.73	>59
eGFR If Africn Am	106		mL/min/1.73	>59
BUN/Creatinine Ratio	9			9 - 23
Sodium	139		mmol/L	134 - 144
Potassium	4.1		mmol/L	3.5 - 5.2
Chloride	109	High	mmol/L	96 - 106
Carbon Dioxide, Total	17	Low	mmol/L	20 - 29
Calcium	8.9		mg/dL	8.7 - 10.2

Normal anion gap metabolic acidosis is caused by the increased loss of bicarbonate from the body, either through the kidney (kidney disease, diuretics, carbonic anhydrase inhibitors like topiramate and acetazolamide) or from the gastrointestinal tract (e.g., severe diarrhea, laxative abuse).

Notice that kidney disease can cause both types of metabolic acidosis.

Important! There are several other possible causes of high anion gap or normal anion gap metabolic acidosis and I have given only a few examples of them here.

Topiramate and metabolic acidosis

You have probably read or heard at some time or the other that some medications used by mental health clinicians (on- or off-label) can cause "metabolic acidosis." Topiramate is probably the most important one of these.

How does topiramate cause metabolic acidosis?

Topiramate inhibits the enzyme carbonic anhydrase that catalyzes the conversion of carbon dioxide plus water into hydrogen and bicarbonate ions. That conversion is necessary to allow the kidneys to excrete hydrogen ions while reabsorbing the bicarbonate ions.

Any risk factors for metabolic acidosis with topiramate?

Metabolic acidosis with topiramate does not seem to be related to the dose of topiramate or to how long the patient has been on topiramate (Mirza et al., 2011).

Short-term clinical features

Topiramate-induced metabolic acidosis may present with:

– Changes on laboratory tests but no symptoms. This is probably the commonest situation

– Non-specific symptoms like fatigue, sleepiness, etc.

– Hyperventilation

– Cardiac arrhythmias

– Acute confusion (so-called "change in mental status")

Long-term risks

In the longer term, metabolic acidosis caused by topiramate can lead to:

– Increased urinary calcium excretion (Barnett et al., 2018)

– Formation of kidney stones (Barnett et al., 2018)

– Osteoporosis (Mirza et al., 2009)

– Growth retardation in children (Mirza et al., 2009)

How to manage metabolic acidosis due to topiramate

We, as mental health clinicians, must not try to manage metabolic acidosis on our own. But, we should have some understanding of it, so that we can intelligently collaborate with the primary care physician or nephrologist.

The best management is, of course, to stop the medication that is causing the metabolic acidosis. If the topiramate is stopped, the metabolic acidosis tends to resolve quickly, even within a week (e.g., Fakhoury et al., 2002).

If that is not possible (unlikely):

– The patient must be regularly monitored for kidney stones. Checking the urine for blood is one way to do that because kidney stones often lead to hematuria. One paper recommended that all children who are put on topiramate should serum electrolytes, urinary calcium, and urinary creatinine at baseline and then "periodically" (Barnett et al., 2018). They also recommended that If the urinary calcium/ creatinine ratio increases to the abnormal range, an ultrasound of the kidney should be done.

– The patient should be told not to follow a ketogenic diet. Some people do that for various reasons.

– The non-mental-health clinician may sometimes prescribe sodium citrate.

References: See https://simpleandpractical.com/side-effects-references

CHAPTER 7: ENDOCRINE GLANDS

HYPERPARATHYROIDISM

Lithium-induced hyperparathyroidism

Clinicians are very aware that lithium can cause hypothyroidism and routinely check thyroid function in patients on lithium. But, should we be routinely screening for lithium-induced hyperparathyroidism?

By the way, don't get mixed up—it is HYPOthyroidism, but HYPERparathyroidism.

How does lithium cause hyperparathyroidism and hypercalcemia?

1. It stimulates the parathyroid glands to release parathyroid hormone

2. It also directly affects the renal tubules to increase the reabsorption of calcium by the kidneys. Make a mental note of this because this will explain why in lithium-induced hyperparathyroidism, usually there is HYPOcalciuria rather than the HYPERcalciuria usually found in primary hyperparathyroidism.

3. It affects the intestine to increase calcium reabsorption.

How common is it?

Lithium-induced hypercalcemia is much more common than we may think! It occurs in approximately 10% of patients on lithium (McKnight et al., 2012).

The prevalence of hypercalcemia in patients on lithium may vary from about 5% (Lally et al., 2013) to about 16% (Twigt et al., 2013), about 18% (Meehan at al., 2015) or even about 25% (Meehan at al., 2018).

Are the prevalence of hypercalcemia and the prevalence of hyperparathyroidism the same thing? Many authors will only call it hyperparathyroidism if the parathyroid hormone level is increased above the normal range. But, we should realize that if the serum calcium level is abnormally elevated, we would expect the parathyroid hormone level to be low in response to that. So, even a normal or high-normal parathyroid hormone level indicates hyperparathyroidism in the face of increased calcium levels.

It is related specifically to lithium. How do we know that?

1. The prevalence of primary hyperparathyroidism in large populations is only 0.1 to 0.2% (Yeh et al., 2013) while increased parathyroid hormone levels are found much more commonly that that in patients who are taking lithium.

2. A meta-analysis of studies found that patients on lithium are much more likely to have hypercalcemia than those on control treatment (McKnight et al., 2012). In a study done after that meta-analysis, patients with bipolar disorder who have hypercalcemia were 13 times more likely to be on lithium than on other medications (Meehan et al., 2018).

Who is at greater risk?

Older age, women (Livinstone and Rampes, 2006), and (maybe) longer duration of treatment with lithium.

What symptoms may occur?

Lithium-induced hyperparathyroidism may be asymptomatic, but as it progresses, symptoms may become apparent.

What symptoms could occur? Have you heard this mnemonic for symptoms may occur with primary hyperparathyroidism (not lithium-induced)—Moans, stones, groans, bones and psychiatric overtones?

Moans–generally not feeling well, weakness, fatigue

Stones–renal stones, nephrocalcinosis, renal impairment

Groans–abdominal pain, dyspepsia, pancreatitis, peptic ulcer disease

Bones–osteopenia, osteoporosis

Psychiatric overtones–mood changes, paranoia, delirium

Also, cardiovascular effects can occur–hypertension, bradycardia, shortened QT interval, asystole (Lienert and Rege, 2008).

Lithium-induced hyperparathyroidism may manifest somewhat differently than primary hyperparathyroidism (Shapiro and Davis, 2015; Livingstone and Rampes, 2006).

Its clinical manifestations may also be milder than those with primary hyperparathyroidism. For example, hypocalciuria rather than hypercalciuria may be present. If so, then the risk of renal stones is likely to be lower. Similarly, lithium-induced hyperparathyroidism may have a lower risk of osteoporosis compared to the risk with primary hyperparathyroidism.

How to screen for lithium-induced hyperparathyroidism

Lithium-induced hypercalcemia or hyperparathyroidism is much more common than we might think. So, we should screen for this potential side effect in ALL patients on lithium.

The most important feature of lithium's effect on the secretion of parathyroid hormone and its additional direct effect on the renal tubules and intestine to increase calcium absorption is hypercalcemia.

It is very important that we understand that the serum calcium may be elevated but the serum parathyroid hormone level may be normal. That is odd, isn't it? We are calling it hyperparathyroidism but the serum parathyroid hormone level may be within the normal range. Many authors will only call it hyperparathyroidism if the parathyroid hormone level is increased above the normal range. But, we should realize that if the serum calcium level is abnormally elevated, we would expect the parathyroid hormone level to be low in response to that. So, even a normal or high-normal parathyroid hormone level indicates a kind of "relative" (my term) hyperparathyroidism when serum calcium is increased.

So, hypercalcemia is what we should screen for rather than checking the serum parathyroid hormone level. The CANMAT guideline for the treatment of bipolar disorder (Yatham et al., 2018) recommends that we should routinely check serum calcium and if that is elevated, to do further testing for hyperparathyroidism. That is, if serum calcium is not elevated, there is no need to do additional tests for hyperparathyroidism. That's the whole point of "screening," right?

How often should serum calcium be checked?

The CANMAT guideline (Yatham et al., 2018) did not recommend a particular frequency and different experts recommend different frequencies for testing serum calcium.

– Some experts recommended that serum calcium should be measured before starting lithium and at least once a year (McKnight et al., 2012; Gitlin, 2016). It should be noted that the once a year is a minimum; more frequent testing is indicated if the serum calcium is abnormal or if the patient has a family history of parathyroid disease (McKnight et al., 2012).

– Other experts have even recommended more frequent testing (every six months or even more frequently).

In my clinical practice, among other tests that I typically order in patients on lithium (or ask for a copy of the results if they were done by someone else), I include:

Yearly–Comprehensive Metabolic Panel

Every six months–Serum lithium level, Basic Metabolic Panel, Thyroid Stimulating Hormone

The basic metabolic panel gives us the serum calcium and the serum creatinine. The comprehensive metabolic panel gives us these as well as serum albumin.

Also check the Vitamin D level

We should also check vitamin D levels in patients on lithium because of two reasons:

1. Serum calcium is closely regulated not only by the parathyroid hormone but also by vitamin D.

2. Low vitamin D levels can increase the secretion of parathyroid hormone (Lehmann and Lee, 2013).

I typically don't check the vitamin D level every year in patients whose level was normal. But, it is amazing how many people have low vitamin D levels!

How to calculate corrected serum calcium

Serum calcium level is of interest to mental health clinicians for several reasons. For example, increased serum calcium (hypercalcemia) is a common side effect of lithium.

Total, Free, and Corrected calcium

You may have heard of correcting serum calcium for the serum albumin level but never clearly understood it. Various authors have explained how to do this in a manner that is unnecessarily complicated, so let me give you a "simple and practical" explanation.

In the blood, half of the calcium is in free, ionized form and the other half is bound to albumin. What we measure in the Basic Metabolic Panel or Comprehensive Metabolic Panel (panels of lab tests very commonly used in the United States), is the total serum calcium, even though the word total is not used in the lab report–it is simply called "serum calcium." It includes both the free, ionized calcium and the calcium that is being transported in the blood bound to albumin.

It is the free, ionized calcium that is biologically active and that we really care about. But, measuring ionized calcium is technically difficult and expensive. So, we usually just measure the (total) serum calcium and serum albumin and use the formula below to "correct" the serum calcium for the serum albumin level.

Corrected serum calcium = serum calcium (total; mg/dL) plus a correction factor

The correction factor to be added to the serum calcium as measured is:

[4 – plasma albumin in g/dL] × 0.8

In the United States, we can think of the Comprehensive Metabolic Panel as a combination of the Basic Metabolic Panel and Hepatic Function Tests. It includes both serum calcium (as part of the Basic Metabolic Panel) and serum albumin (as part of the Hepatic Function Tests).

If the serum calcium is on the higher side of normal, we should look at the serum albumin. If the serum albumin is abnormally low, then the corrected serum calcium level may be abnormally high even if it looks like it is in the normal range.

To understand this, let's look at this lab result from one of my patients who is on lithium.

```
Comp. Metabolic Panel (14)
Glucose                   95          mg/dL         65 - 99
BUN                       12          mg/dL          6 - 20
Creatinine              1.22          mg/dL       0.76 - 1.27
eGFR If NonAfricn Am      81      mL/min/1.73          >59
eGFR If Africn Am         94      mL/min/1.73          >59
BUN/Creatinine Ratio      10                         9 - 20
Sodium                   138          mmol/L       134 - 144
Potassium                4.3          mmol/L       3.5 - 5.2
Chloride                  99          mmol/L        96 - 106
Carbon Dioxide, Total     24          mmol/L        18 - 29
Calcium                  9.9          mg/dL        8.7 - 10.2
Protein, Total           7.3          g/dL         6.0 - 8.5
Albumin                  4.8          g/dL         3.5 - 5.5
Globulin, Total          2.5          g/dL         1.5 - 4.5
A/G Ratio                1.9                       1.2 - 2.2
Bilirubin, Total         1.2          mg/dL        0.0 - 1.2
Alkaline Phosphatase      63          IU/L          39 - 117
AST (SGOT)                19          IU/L           0 - 40
ALT (SGPT)                25          IU/L           0 - 44
```

The serum calcium, 9.9 mg/dL is within the normal range shown for this lab (8.7 to 10.2 mg/dL), but on the higher side of that range. So, I would check to make sure his serum albumin is not low and in this case, it is not. But, what if everything remained the same but his serum albumin was a bit low, say 3.0 g/dL, which is not even extremely low?

The correction factor that we would add to the serum calcium as measured would be $(4 - 3) \times 0.8 = 0.8$. That is, his corrected serum calcium would have been 10.7, which would be higher than the normal range.

Now, our astute readers will soon figure out from the formula that:

– If the serum albumin in 4, then we add nothing to the measured serum calcium to correct it

– If the serum albumin is anything less than 4, even within the normal range for serum albumin, we need to add something to the measured serum calcium to get the corrected serum calcium.

– If the serum albumin is anything more than 4, even within the normal range for serum albumin, we need to subtract something to the measured serum calcium to get the corrected serum calcium.

So, calculating a corrected serum calcium is most important when the serum albumin is less than 4 g/dL and the serum calcium is on the higher side of the normal range. But, if we want to track gradual change over the years in the corrected serum calcium, then we would have to calculate the corrected value for each year.

Lithium-induced hyperparathyroidism: Management

The treatment of lithium-induced hyperparathyroidism in generally similar to that for hyperparathyroidism due to any other reason. But, let's look at what our options are.

Wait and watch (just monitor)

If the lithium-induced hyperparathyroidism is mild and asymptomatic, we can just wait and watch (Gitlin, 2016) to see if it gets worse or stays clinically unimportant.

Taper off the lithium?

If the hyperparathyroidism is clinically significant, we should strongly consider changing from lithium to another medication.

After stopping the lithium, it is possible that the hypercalcemia may resolve, as happened in one published case (Khandwal and Van Uum, 2006). But, lithium-induced hyperparathyroidism may not resolve in many cases even after stopping the lithium (Sloand and Shelly, 2006).

(*Optional to read:* In one study, the elevations in serum calcium did not improve after being off lithium for a mean of 8.5 (range 4 to 16) weeks (Bendz et al., 1996). Of course, in that study, we don't know whether longer periods off lithium could have led to resolution of lithium-induced hyperparathyroidism.)

Note: It may still be a good idea to stop lithium if possible because if lithium is continued after surgical excision of a parathyroid adenoma, this may lead to multiglandular disease (Järhult et al., 2010).

In the cases in which the serum calcium does normalize after stopping lithium, it is not clear how likely it is that this will happen or how long this might take.

Due to the uncertainties discussed above, if the hypercalcemia is severe enough, even if the lithium has been stopped, the endocrinologist may suggest proceeding to active treatment of the hypercalcemia without waiting too long.

As mental health clinicians we will not treat lithium-induced hyperparathyroidism ourselves, but we do need to know a bit about the treatment options so that we can discuss them with our patients if the need arises.

Surgical treatment

The main treatment of hyperparathyroidism in general is surgery. Surgical treatment for has also been used specifically for lithium-induced hyperparathyroidism as well (Carchman et al., 2008; Szalat et al., 2009; Marti et al., 2012; Meehan et al., 2018).

What kind of surgery? Each person has four parathyroid glands. In about a quarter of patients with lithium-induced hyperparathyroidism, there is multiglandular disease (Carchman et al., 2008). In such cases, it will probably be necessary to remove most, but not all, of the parathyroid tissue ("subtotal" parathyroidectomy).

But, in three-fourths of cases of lithium-induced hyperparathyroidism, there is a single adenoma (Carchman et al., 2008). In such cases, localized surgery to remove the adenoma is done.

But, it is not clear what the longer-term results of surgery for lithium-induced hyperparathyroidism are. Unfortunately, they may be disappointing in many cases (Järhult et al., 2010). This is probably because it is very hard for the surgeon to find and remove all parathyroid gland tissue and activity of the remaining parathyroid tissue may lead to the serum calcium going up again (Dixon et al., 2018).

Cinacalcet

What if parathyroidectomy is not successful or the patient is not suited for surgery due to any reason? Or if it is absolutely essential that the lithium be continued even though the patient has developed hypercalcemia/hyperparathyroidism? What then?

In the parathyroid gland (and the kidneys and other tissues), a feedback loop is present. When extracellular calcium acts on the calcium-sensing receptor in the parathyroid gland, it leads to activation of this receptor and to a decrease in parathyroid hormone secretion. It is like the calcium saying to the parathyroid gland—"We have enough calcium, there is no need for so much parathyroid hormone." This is similar to thyroid hormone acting on the pituitary gland and turning down the release of thyroid stimulating hormone by the pituitary.

While lithium probably causes hypercalcemia by several mechanisms—and these are not well known—it is believed that one of the mechanisms is antagonism of the activity of the calcium-sensing receptor (Brown, 1981).

Cinacalcet (brand name Sensipar®, developed by Amgen, Inc) is a medication that increases the sensitivity of the calcium-sensing receptors in the parathyroid gland to activation by extracellular calcium, and so, it reduces the release of parathyroid hormone. That is why, cinacalcet is said to be "calcimimetic"; that is, it mimics the action of calcium. Cinacalcet is known to be an effective treatment for both primary and secondary hyperparathyroidism.

Does cinacalcet also work for lithium-induced hyperparathyroidism?

While as of April 2019, I am not aware of any clinical trial of cinacalcet specifically for lithium-induced hyperparathyroidism, in several published case reports, cinacalcet was effective for lithium-induced hyperparathyroidism (e.g., Sloand and Shelly, 2006; Gregoor et al., 2007; Dixon et al., 2018).

Treatment with cinacalcet may be particularly useful in cases in which it is important to not stop the lithium (e.g., Dixon et al., 2018).

HYPERPROLACTINEMIA

Can buspirone cause increased prolactin or galactorrhea?

Can medication A cause side effect X?

This is such a common situation. A patient reports a new symptom or sign and asks whether it may be due to a particular medication. How would we try to answer the question about whether medication A is known to sometimes cause side effect X? Let's look at what we might do, starting with the simplest options and proceeding to more complicated options only if needed.

Since we know that galactorrhea may be caused by elevated prolactin levels (it can also occur with normal prolactin levels), we should search for both terms—galactorrhea and prolactin.

Our adverse effect handouts

The SIMPLEST option is to go to https://simpleandpractical.com/aehandouts and look at the document listing common and less common potential "side effects" of various psychotropic medications. You can find the link to these documents on our website by going to the Resources menu at the top of any page on the website.

In looking at the handout on potential side effects of buspirone, we don't see the words "galactorrhea" or "prolactin". This tells us that elevated prolactin or galactorrhea is not among the common, well-known side effects of buspirone.

The Prescribing Information

The next step is to find the official Prescribing Information (also called the Product Label) for buspirone. To do this, we Google the words "BuSpar PI" or "buspirone PI". BuSpar is the trade name and buspirone is the generic name; either will work.

We can then easily search the Prescribing Information document for the words "prolactin" and "galactorrhea" by using Control+F on a PC computer or Command+F on a Mac computer. When we do this in the buspirone Prescribing Information, we don't find the word "prolactin" anywhere in the document but we do find the word "galactorrhea".

In listing all the adverse events that were associated with buspirone, the Prescribing Information lists "galactorrhea" as a "rare" adverse event in patients on buspirone. ("Rare" events were those occurring in less than 0.1% of patients on the medication.)

Micromedex

I also looked up the adverse effects of buspirone in Micromedex, a subscription database to which I have free access through the university where I teach. It noted:

"Hyperprolactinemia

a) Dose-dependent increases in serum prolactin have been described with busPIRone"

PubMed

I looked up the reference cited in Micromedex and a related one (Meltzer et al., 1983; Meltzer et al., 1982) on PubMed and found the following statements:

"…preclinical studies have shown that [buspirone] produces effects consistent with both a dopamine agonist and antagonist."

"In a double-blind placebo-controlled study using eight normal male volunteers, buspirone (30, 60, and 90 mg) produced a dose-related increase in [prolactin] levels 60-180 minutes later…"

"The apparent increase in [prolactin] secretion was dose dependent…"

Clinical recommendations

1. If we are faced with a situation of galactorrhea associated with any psychotropic medication, it would be a good idea to measure a serum prolactin level before doing anything else. This is important for establishing what is going on and may be important later on.

2. We should also remember that many psychotropic medications can cause elevated prolactin and/or galactorrhea, including antipsychotics and antidepressants. If more that one medication was started around the same time, it may be unclear which medication caused the side effect. Or, it could be due to a combination of factors.

How to measure and interpret serum prolactin

Prolactin levels are important to mental health professionals for several reasons:

1. Some psychiatric medications can increase prolactin levels (e.g., antipsychotics)

2. Elevated prolactin levels can be a cause of sexual dysfunction

3. Elevated prolactin levels may be a clue that the person's headaches and visual problems are due to a pituitary tumor
How to measure serum prolactin

The following FOUR instructions need to be given to patients to make sure that we don't get a false estimate of serum prolactin.

1. Time of the day

Serum prolactin levels vary over the day. It is recommended that the level should be measured in the morning, preferably a few hours after waking up.

2. Fasting

The person should be fasting.

3. Exercise

Exercise can falsely elevate serum prolactin. The person should be advised to avoid strenuous exercise on the morning of the test and to rest for 20 to 30 minutes before the level is drawn.

4. Stress/ anxiety

Stress and anxiety can also lead to falsely elevated serum prolactin levels. If the prolactin level is high (even two to three times normal), we should ask whether the person has a needle phobia, had a difficult venipuncture, or was particularly stressed or anxious at the time the blood was drawn. Attempts should be made to repeat the serum prolactin under better conditions. These could include a more experienced person doing the blood draw, distracting the person, or use of lidocaine ointment at the venipuncture site prior to drawing blood.

Symptoms

We noted above that we should ask if the patient had exercised strenuously or was under stress at the time that the blood was drawn for measurement of serum prolactin.

In addition, we should ask patients a few questions to get an idea of the clinical significance of the elevated serum prolactin and to get a clue to its possible etiology. It may be easier to remember what to ask by going from one part of the body to another as follows:

In the head: headaches, visual disturbances. Both of these could suggest a pituitary tumor.

In the breasts: gynecomastia in men, galactorrhea (for both females and males). It should be obvious but one author (Levy, 2014) reminds us that we ask about galactorrhea, not examine the patient for it.

In the genital area: amenorrhea, infertility, sexual dysfunction

All over the body: hirsutism (for possible polycystic ovarian syndrome, which could be the cause of the elevated prolactin). We should ask the patient rather than relying on what we see since women with hirsutism generally actively remove the hair and so the presence of hirsutism may be missed (Levy, 2014). Polycystic ovarian syndrome is commonly associated with depression and anxiety symptoms. We, as mental health professionals, need to do a better job of identifying PCOS in our patients.

Importantly, get a complete list of the medications that the person is taking.

Further laboratory tests

These should be done to rule out certain causes of elevated prolactin. Here are some that the mental health professional can order rather than requiring that the patient see a specialist first.

1. Importantly, check TSH since hypothyroidism leads to elevated prolactin

2. If there is any chance of pregnancy or ectopic pregnancy, check a pregnancy test.

3. Serum creatinine (renal insufficiency can lead to elevated prolactin)

4. If polycystic ovarian syndrome is suspected, check total and free testosterone level.

Normal values

The normal values for prolactin may vary a bit between laboratories. The following values are suggested by medlineplus.gov:

Males: less than 20 ng/mL (425 mIU/L)

Nonpregnant females: 5 to 40 ng/mL (106 to 850 mIU/L)

Pregnant women: 80 to 400 ng/mL (1,700 to 8,500 mIU/L)

When to worry (or not)

Serious: If the serum prolactin is significantly high (e.g., greater than 200 ng/mL) and/or the person has persistent headaches or visual disturbances, we should refer the person to a specialist for diagnostic imaging of the sella turcica to look for a pituitary adenoma. This is very important to remember.

Less serious: Stress and sleep disturbance can lead to elevated serum prolactin. So, if the elevation of serum prolactin in mild, we could wait and retest before deciding how to proceed.

Management of hyperprolactinemia

Prolactin level

Severe galactorrhea requires measuring the prolactin level, which is otherwise not required. If it is greater than 200 ng/ ml, an MRI may be in order to rule out a pituitary adenoma.

Reduce the dose, if possible

It is common and sensible to say that, if possible, we should reduce the dose of any medication that is causing any adverse effects. But, reducing the dose usually increases the risk of relapse of the condition being treated. So, this is easier said than done.

Also, based on a small sample, there is a suggestion that risperidone-induced hyperprolactinemia may not be clearly dose-related (Daniels et al., 2011). But, I am not yet confident that this is true.

Switching the antipsychotic

It is unusual to be unable to switch from risperidone to one of the other 11 atypical antipsychotics. That implies that the patient had either failed to respond to or to tolerate all the other second-generation antipsychotics.

Adding aripiprazole

But if that is the case, I usually add aripiprazole, a prolactin-lowering dopamine partial agonist, in doses titrated up to 20 mg/ day to offset the hyperprolactinemia. Several published studies also support this.

Not only is the dose important, but also the duration of treatment with aripiprazole. It may take two to three weeks to reverse severe galactorrhea like this.

I have had success by adding aripiprazole the majority of the time. There are many published studies (not just case reports) of this approach to managing hyperprolactinemia.

Note: When aripiprazole is added to an antipsychotic to treat hyperprolactinemia, we should titrate up to 15 or 20 mg per day AND try it for at least two to three weeks before concluding that it did not work.]

Bromocriptine

Before the advent of partial agonists, I used bromocriptine. Just as we sometimes used amantadine in the past for extrapyramidal symptoms (instead of benztropine) and avoided psychotic relapses by titrating it slowly, the same is done with bromocriptine. Relapse is unlikely if the antipsychotic dose is adequate.

THYROID DYSFUNCTION

An introduction to lithium-induced hypothyroidism

Lithium use can be associated with several different types of thyroid problems. Some of these are very common! The types of problems that can occur include:

– *Clinical hypothyroidism* (clinical symptoms, elevated thyroid-stimulating hormone or TSH, low T4)

– *Subclinical hypothyroidism* (no clinical symptoms, elevated thyroid-stimulating hormone or TSH, normal T4)

– *Goiter* (enlarged thyroid gland with decreased, normal, or increased thyroid function). Thyroid function may be normal in these patients because the gland has hypertrophied enough to be able to produce adequate amounts of thyroid hormone.

– Rarely, hyperthyroidism (Livingstone and Rampes, 2006)

Note: Lithium does not cause thyroid nodules, so if a thyroid nodule is found, another cause should be looked for.

Mechanism

Lithium affects thyroid function through effects on several different steps in thyroid gland function ranging from the uptake of iodine to release of thyroid hormones into the blood (McKnight et al., 2012; Gitlin, 2016; Livingstone and Rampes, 2006).

(Optional to read: One author states that the main mechanism by which lithium causes hypothyroidism is believed to be inhibition of release of thyroid hormone from the thyroid gland but other mechanisms may also be involved; Gitlin, 2016).

Symptoms

The symptoms of lithium-induced hyperthyroidism (an example of secondary hypothyroidism) are the same as those in primary hypothyroidism.

How common is lithium-induced hypothyroidism?

Clinical hypothyroidism

In this, there are clinical symptoms of hypothyroidism, elevated thyroid stimulating hormone or TSH, and low T4.

The incidence of clinical hypothyroidism in patients on lithium has been reported to be between 8 to 19%, compared to only 0.5% to 1.8% in the general population (Kleiner et al., 1999).

So, let's say about 10% incidence of clinical hypothyroidism, which is about ten times more than in the general population.

Subclinical hypothyroidism

In this, there are no clinical symptoms of hypothyroidism, elevated thyroid stimulating hormone or TSH, and normal T4.

An incidence of up to 23% was described in an older review (Kleiner et al., 1999), but a later study reported that 36% of patients started on lithium developed either an elevated TSH or an abnormal free thyroxine index (FTI; Fagiolini et al., 2006).

So, let's say between a quarter and one-third of patients on lithium develop subclinical hypothyroidism.

Goiter

When the size of the thyroid gland was carefully evaluated in one study using ultrasound, a goiter (enlarged thyroid gland) was present in about 50% of patients on lithium (Bauer et al., 2007).

What are the risk factors for lithium-induced hypothyroidism?

The following factors increase the chances that the person will subsequently develop lithium-induced hypothyroidism:

– Female sex. Females are up to five times more likely to develop lithium-induced hypothyroidism (Livingstone and Rampes, 2006). This may be due to females being much more likely to be positive for antithyroid antibodies (Kraszewska et al. 2015; Shine et al. 2015).

– Age greater than 50 years

– Starting lithium in middle age (Johnston and Eagles, 1999)

– Predisposition to autoimmune thyroiditis. This includes being positive for antithyroid antibodies (eight times greater risk, Bocchetta et al., 1992, 2001, 2007)

– Family history of hypothyroidism in first-degree relatives (Kibrige et al. 2013).

– Longer duration of treatment. The risk if cumulative and increases over the years of treatment.

– Higher baseline TSH (Henry, 2002; Gracious et al., 2004)

– Higher lithium levels (Gracious et al., 2004)

When and how often should we screen for lithium-induced hypothyroidism?

To screen for possible thyroid dysfunction due to lithium, serum thyroid-stimulating hormone (TSH) should be checked:

– At baseline

– At three months (because hypothyroidism often develops early on)

– At six months

– Then, every six to twelve months. I aim for every six months since often there is a delay due to one reason or another.

What about checking free T4?

Experts disagree about whether free T4 and antithyroid antibodies should be checked even if TSH is normal.

While we can order a combination test for TSH plus free T4 (see on

Labcorp's website), I typically order only TSH to screen for lithium-induced hypothyroidism.

Then, if the TSH comes back abnormally high (or maybe even if it is at the higher side of the normal range), then definitely we need to check for free T4, which helps us to differentiate between:

– Subclinical hypothyroidism (elevated TSH, normal free T4, no clinical symptoms of hypothyroidism), and

– Clinical hypothyroidism (elevated TSH, low free T4, usually with clinical symptoms of hypothyroidism).

Antithyroid antibodies

Antithyroid antibodies suggest autoimmune thyroiditis. What is the significance in patients treated with lithium of being positive for antithyroid antibodies at baseline (Kleiner et al., 1999)?

1. They are more likely to develop hypothyroidism

2. The hypothyroidism is likely to be more severe

3. The hypothyroidism may not resolve even if the lithium is stopped.

But (Kleiner et al., 1999):

– Not everyone with antithyroid antibodies at baseline develops hypothyroidism while on lithium

– Patients negative for antithyroid antibodies at baseline may also develop hypothyroidism while on lithium.

I don't check antithyroid antibodies at baseline or follow up unless the TSH is abnormally elevated. I also asked two of the top bipolar disorders experts in the world and they both said that's what they do too.

If the TSH is abnormally elevated and we want to check for antithyroid antibodies, which ones should we order?

The two antithyroid antibodies that are commonly tested for together are:

– Thyroid Peroxidase (TPO) antibodies (see on Labcorp's website)

– Thyroglobulin antibody (see on Labcorp's website)

Both antibodies should be tested for, so it is more convenient to order "Thyroid antibodies"(see on Labcorp's website), which combines testing for both of them.

If antithyroid antibodies are positive, I recommend referring the patient to an endocrinologist (or primary care physician if seeing an endocrinologist is not feasible) for further evaluation and treatment.

Other tests?

Some experts recommend an ultrasound of the thyroid gland (as noted by Gitlin, 2006) but most of us don't order that. When evaluated by ultrasound, the thyroid gland is enlarged in up to 50% of patients on lithium. This is because the elevated TSH leads to thyroid hypertrophy that, at least initially, maintains normal thyroid hormone levels.

How should lithium-induced hypothyroidism be managed?

In this section, let's discuss what we should do if the thyroid-stimulating hormone (TSH) level was normal before starting lithium but comes back abnormally high (suggesting a decrease in thyroid function) while the person is being treated with lithium?

First, recheck TSH and check free T4 and antithyroid antibodies

We should not overreact to a single value of elevated TSH. TSH can sometimes be temporarily increased due to acute illness or stress. So, we should recheck the TSH a few weeks later and also check free T4 and antithyroid antibodies at that time.

If the repeat TSH comes back high again and free T4 is decreased, the patient has clinical hypothyroidism and needs treatment with thyroid hormone.

But what if the repeat TSH comes back high and the free T4 is normal and antithyroid antibodies are negative? This is subclinical hypothyroidism and is the most common scenario.

Continue lithium or stop it?

If the person has had a good response to lithium treatment, the occurrence of lithium-induced hypothyroidism is not by itself a reason to stop lithium (Yatham et al., 2018; Gitlin, 2016). Let's keep in mind that hypothyroidism is relatively easy to treat by giving thyroid hormone and that for some patients, lithium is a uniquely effective medication.

But if the lithium has not been very helpful or side effects other than hypothyroidism are present, a decision may be taken to stop the lithium. We should remember to not stop lithium abruptly but to taper it off over several weeks.

If the lithium is stopped, will the hypothyroidism be reversed? That is the 64-dollar question, isn't it? We don't have a reliable answer to this question from systematic research, but it is believed that in many cases, the hypothyroidism may resolve if the lithium is stopped (Kleiner et al., 1999; Gitlin, 2016). We may assume that this is more likely if antithyroid antibodies are negative, the TSH elevation was relatively mild, and the hypothyroidism was identified early on due to careful monitoring, but none of this has been systematically researched.

TSH between 5 and 10 mIU/L

If the TSH is between 4 and 10 mIU/L, free T4 is normal, antithyroid antibodies are negative, and the patient does not have symptoms that may be related to hypothyroidism (weight gain, depression, cognitive dulling, fatigue, lethargy, treatment-resistance, rapid cycling, etc.), then we could just monitor more frequently, e.g., after one month and then every three months (Kleiner et al., 1999; Livingstone and Rampes, 2006).

But if there are clinical symptoms, thyroid hormone treatment should be considered.

TSH more than 10 mIU/L

While there is controversy over this, many experts think that such patients are at high risk of progressing to clinical hypothyroidism and should be treated even if free T4 is normal and there are no clinical symptoms (Kleiner et al., 1999; Gitlin, 2006). In other words, subclinical hypothyroidism should usually be treated if TSH is more than 10 mIU/L.

References: See https://simpleandpractical.com/side-effects-references

CHAPTER 8: EYES

BLURRED VISION

Psychotropic medications and blurred vision

Blurred vision is a relatively common potential side effect of several psychotropic medications.

Here's why it happens, how the patient should be evaluated, and what we can do about it.

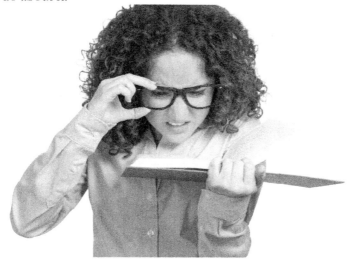

How psychotropic medications cause blurred vision

Knowing just the basics of how psychotropic medications cause blurred vision will guide us in how to evaluate and treat patients with this side effect.

Psychotropic medications cause blurred vision through a combination of:

1. Mydriasis (dilation of the pupil), and

2. Cycloplegia (paralysis of the ciliary body of the eye that is responsible for accommodation or the ability to see near objects).

What is the ciliary body and what does it have to do with blurred vision?

The ciliary body of the eye is a circular muscle that surrounds the lens of the eye. The lens is usually kept stretched wide and thinned out due to the elastic pull of the eyeball. But, when the ciliary body contracts, it squeezes the lens and makes it thicker. This increases the refractive power of the eye. This process is called accommodation and is what allows us to be able to focus on near objects.

Medications with anticholinergic effects paralyze the ciliary body; this paralysis is called cycloplegia. When cycloplegia occurs, the patient has difficulty seeing near objects. This is the same problem that we have when we age and need reading glasses (sigh!). But, this problem with aging, called presbyopia, which literally means "old eye", is due to a different reason. It is not due to a change in the ciliary body but because the lens of the eye becomes stiffer with age and has difficulty becoming thicker in order to be able to focus on near objects. Younger readers: Don't worry; you'll get there too!

How do psychotropic medications cause dilation of the pupil and cycloplegia?

1. Cholinergic (parasympathetic) nerves supply both the sphincter pupillae muscle that constricts the pupil and the ciliary body that allows us to see near objects (McDougal and Gamlin, 2015).

Knowing these facts explains why medications with anticholinergic effects are particularly problematic in terms of causing blurred vision. They cause blurred vision by causing both dilation of the pupil and loss of accommodation. These medications include anticholinergics (e.g., benztropine), tricyclic antidepressants (in about one-third of patients; Richa and Yazbek, 2010), and low-potency antipsychotics.

What about other psychotropic medications—ones that don't have any significant anticholinergic effects?

2. Sympathetic nerves supply the dilator pupillae muscle that, as the name suggests, leads to dilation of the pupil (McDougal and Gamlin, 2015).

3. Also, the parts of the brain involved in the control of dilation and constriction of the pupil get input from fibers that release dopamine, norepinephrine, histamine, or serotonin (McDougal and Gamlin, 2015). Increased activity of dopaminergic, noradrenergic, and serotonergic inputs to these centers causes dilation of the pupil (McDougal and Gamlin, 2015).

This is why antidepressants like serotonin-norepinephrine reuptake inhibitors (SNRIs) and SSRIs that don't have significant anticholinergic activity can also cause blurred vision—by causing dilation of the pupil. For example, SSRIs cause blurred vision in 2 to 10% of patients (Richa and Yazbek, 2010) and "abnormal vision" was reported by 4% of patients treated with venlafaxine in clinical trials (Prescribing Information).

4. While blurred vision with second-generation antidepressants is benign in most cases, since these antidepressants can cause mydriasis (dilation of the pupil), they can precipitate narrow-angle glaucoma, a very serious side effect, in predisposed patients. In many such patients, blurred vision can be an initial presenting symptom, e.g., with topiramate (Richa and Yazbek, 2010).

Next, let's discuss what to ask and look for in a patient on a psychotropic medication who is complaining of blurred vision to help determine what is going on and to decide whether the person may have a more serious underlying problem.

Evaluation

It is very important to ask about other symptoms that may be present along with the blurred vision because these may provide clues as to why there is blurred vision. These additional symptoms may also suggest the presence of other, potentially very serious, eye problems.

Some expected symptoms

– Blurred vision worse on trying to read or look at near objects? This suggests a problem with accommodation, which is to be expected when blurred vision is due to the anticholinergic effects of a medication.

– Other anticholinergic side effects? E.g., dry mouth, constipation. These would support the assessment that the blurred vision is due to anticholinergic effects.

–Pupil dilated? Dilation of the pupil may be found with several different medications including those with anticholinergic, adrenergic, or serotonergic effects.

–Photophobia? When blurring of vision is due to abnormal dilation of the pupil, the patient may also notice an increased sensitivity to light.

Symptoms that are concerning

– Irritation/ redness/ tearing in the eye? This may suggest dryness of the eye, problems with contact lenses, etc. If redness of the conjunctiva and tearing are present, these are causes for concern.

– Severe eye pain? This suggests the possibility of acute angle-closure glaucoma and should be considered to be a medical emergency.

– Recent decrease in night vision? If this is present, it may suggest potentially serious retinal disease.

– Papilledema? This refers to swelling of the optic nerve due to increased intracranial pressure. If along with the blurred vision, the patient also has impairment of vision (which may be episodic), vomiting, or headache, it is possible that the patient has papilledema. An ophthalmological examination of the fundus of the eye should be recommended on an urgent basis.

Some questions to ask in evaluating a patient with blurred vision

I started one of my patients on escitalopram 10 mg half tablet in the morning after breakfast; increase to one tablet in the morning after 4 days if tolerated.

A week later, he sent me a secure message through the electronic medical record that I use for my private practice. He said that he had developed mild blurred vision since starting the escitalopram. His other medications had remained the same. He reminded me that he had also developed blurred vision when I had previously prescribed him desvenlafaxine.

What would you do in this situation?

He had an appointment to see me in another week. I assumed that it was a side effect of the escitalopram. SSRIs cause blurred vision in 2 to 10% of patients (Richa and Yazbek, 2010). Because of that, I did not think it was appropriate to tell him to call his primary care doctor or to see an ophthalmologist. The side effect is typically benign, so I did not think that an urgent evaluation by me or anyone else was essential either. But, it was very important that I not assume too much.

So, I responded to his message by sending him some questions in the electronic medical record. Here are the questions and the reasons for asking them. (I sent him only the questions, not the reasons why I was asking them):

To identify cycloplegia (paralysis of accommodation of the eye) as the reason for the blurred vision

– Is the blurred vision worse on trying to read or look at near objects?

– Does wearing reading glasses help the blurred vision?

My patient said "Yes" to both of these questions. Note that using reading glasses is an easy way to deal with medication-induced blurred vision while waiting for it to decrease on its own.

My patient said "No" to all the other questions.

To assess if excessive dilation of the pupil and impairment of pupillary constriction are present

– Have you become more intolerant to bright light than in the past?

To try to rule out dryness or infection of the eyes

– Do you have irritation in one or both eyes?

– Do you have redness in one or both eyes?

– Do you have tearing in one or both eyes?

To try to rule out serious possibilities like narrow-angle glaucoma

– Do you have pain in one or both eyes?

To try to rule out retinal disease

– Have you had a recent decrease in night vision?

To try to rule out papilledema

– Has your vision become worse—intermittently or continuously?

– Have you had vomiting recently?

-. Did you develop a new headache recently?

To assess if the blurred vision is an anticholinergic side effect

This did not apply to my patient who was started on escitalopram because it does not have any significant anticholinergic activity. But, we can also ask some questions about symptoms of anticholinergic side effects if the medication associated with the development of blurred vision is known to have anticholinergic side effects. For example:

– Do you also have dry mouth?

– Do you also have constipation?

– Do you think you are sweating less than normal?

GLAUCOMA

Psychotropic medications and glaucoma

Several psychotropic medications have been associated with acute angle-closure glaucoma, which is a medical emergency and can be associated with loss of vision. These include:

1. Antidepressants: bupropion, SSRIs (especially, paroxetine), mirtazapine, venlafaxine, tricyclic antidepressants (TCAs), etc.

2. Antipsychotics, e.g., clozapine, olanzapine

3. Others, e.g., topiramate

Angle closure glaucoma is also called narrow-angle glaucoma. The "angle" refers to the angle between the cornea and the iris. The other type of glaucoma is called open-angle glaucoma.

What are the symptoms of an attack of acute angle-closure glaucoma?

These may include:

– sudden onset of severe pain in the eye

– redness and swelling of the eye

– tearing from the eye

– impairment of vision

– photophobia

Acute angle-closure glaucoma is a true emergency because if not treated immediately, it can result in permanent blindness.

Who is at higher risk?

Glaucoma precipitated by psychotropic medications is, of course, uncommon. But it is important that if we come across a patient who is at high-risk, we are ready to realize this.

What is the single more important thing to ask about?

Persons with a family history of acute angle-closure glaucoma are TEN times more likely to develop acute angle-closure glaucoma. So, we should routinely ask patients whether they or any family member has ever had glaucoma or increased pressure in the eye.

Demographics

The person at highest risk is:

– Elderly

– Female

– Of Asian, Indian, Hispanic, or Inuit origin

To remember this, you can think of any person whom you know who fits this description. For example, in my case, my mother is an elderly female of Indian origin and can help me to remember the risk factors for angle-closure glaucoma. (Only as a mnemonic aid—she is not on an antidepressant and never had glaucoma.)

Factors related to the eye

– Farsighted (technically called hyperopia or hypermetropia)

– Small eye (technically called nanophthalmos)

– Structure of the eye (only an ophthalmologist would be able to evaluate these): shallow depth of the anterior chamber of the eye, anatomically narrow angle.

Medications

Medications can precipitate acute angle closure glaucoma due to many different reasons. Most importantly, medications that make the pupils dilate can precipitate this kind of glaucoma. When the pupils dilate, the angle of the eye gets further blocked. For example, bupropion, SSRIs, SNRIs, etc all can cause pupillary dilation.

References: See https://simpleandpractical.com/side-effects-references

CHAPTER 9: GASTROINTESTINAL TRACT

CONSTIPATION

Constipation is one of the most important potential side effects of clozapine and is the result of clozapine-induced gastrointestinal hypomotility (CIGH). Let's start with some basic facts about it:

— Constipation occurs in at least 30% of patients on clozapine, perhaps more (Sagy et al., 2014).

— Patients on clozapine are much more likely to have constipation than patients taking other antipsychotics (Shirazi et al., 2016).

— It typically occurs within the first few months after starting clozapine (Chougule et al., 2018).

— Constipation is believed to be due to the anticholinergic and antiserotonergic (5-HT3) effects of clozapine (Sagy et al., 2014). Clozapine has the strongest anticholinergic activity among the second-generation antipsychotics. The anticholinergic side effects of clozapine generally correlate with its serum levels.

Potential complications

The constipation may lead to (listed in no particular order; Sagy et al., 2014):

— Fecal impaction, which may be very serious (Rege and Lafferty, 2008).

— Rectal prolapse

— Bowel obstruction

— Paralytic ileus (Ingimarsson et al., 2018)

— Megacolon

– Gastrointestinal ischemia and bowel necrosis

– Intraabdominal sepsis (Oke et al., 2015)

– Death (Levin et al., 2002; Hibbard et al., 2009). Readers may be surprised to know that three times more patients on clozapine die from complications of constipation than from agranulocytosis (Ellis et al., 2006; Sagy et al., 2014). Up to 30% of severe cases may die.

Evaluation of clozapine-induced constipation

Because clozapine-induced constipation is so common, patients who are started on clozapine should be asked routinely, regularly, and specifically about constipation, starting even before the medication is started.

The number of bowel movements per week should be noted down and tracked—especially during the first few months.

Management of clozapine-induced constipation

Much of what will be discussed about the management of clozapine-induced constipation also applies to the management of constipation due to other causes. But, there are a few important points about clozapine-induced constipation:

– Since clozapine-induced constipation can progress to the serious consequences discussed above, it is very important to take constipation in patients on clozapine very seriously and to treat it aggressively.

– We should also keep in mind that patients with schizophrenia may not report constipation or abdominal pain reliably either due to their illness or because they may have abnormalities in the perception of pain. This can put them in danger of developing life-threatening bowel obstruction by the time their caregivers realize that something is wrong.

– If there is significant abdominal pain or distention, vomiting, etc., bowel obstruction may be present. This should be treated as a medical emergency and the patient should be sent to the emergency room for evaluation.

Basic (level 1) measures

To repeat: Much of what will be discussed about the management of clozapine-induced constipation also applies to the management of constipation due to other causes.

To start with, here are some simple, basic things that can be done.

1. It may be a good idea to ask all patients started on clozapine to preventively increase their a) fiber intake, b) water intake, and c) physical activity.

Note: When fiber intake is increased, it is important to also increase fluid intake to prevent bowel obstruction. Also, patients should be told to increase their fiber intake only gradually because fiber can cause bloating and flatulence when transit through the intestines is slow, as it is in persons on clozapine.

2. Also, if the patient is on another anticholinergic medications (hopefully not), the anticholinergic medication should be tapered and stopped if at all possible because the anticholinergic medications will make constipation more likely in persons on clozapine and make it more severe if it is already present.

3. We should tell patients that bowel motility is greater in the morning and after meals. So, after breakfast may be the best time to try.

4. We should also tell patients that they should not strain to pass stools because this can lead to other problems like hemorrhoids or even rectal prolapse.

5. At the first sign of constipation, a stool softener like docusate (brand name Colace) should be started. Docusate is available over-the-counter and a typical dose for adults is 100 mg one to three times a day.

Intermediate (level 2) measures

Early use of laxatives should be considered. Here are some points to keep in mind regarding the use of laxatives for clozapine-induced constipation.

– While much of what we are discussing about the management of clozapine-induced constipation also applies to the management of constipation due to other causes, bulk-forming laxatives, e.g., psyllium (brand name Metamucil) or methylcellulose (brand name Citrucel), which are good choices for other types of constipation, are not recommended for clozapine-induced constipation because they don't work well for slow-transit constipation like the one caused by clozapine.

– One good choice is an osmotic laxative like polyethylene glycol (PEG) 3350 (brand name Miralax). The dose of PEG is 17 g per day. It is available as a powder in a bottle with a cap that allows measurement of 17 g or as packets of pre-measured 17 g. In either case, the powder should be taken by mixing it into 4 to 8 ounces of any fluid (hot or cold).

– Lactulose is another option for an osmotic laxative but is less effective than polyethylene glycol (Lee-Robichaud et al., 2010), but we should remember that it takes up to 3 days to work.

– A stimulant laxative like bisacodyl (brand name Dulcolax) or senna is also commonly used. Bisacodyl is available over the counter. The recommended dose for adolescents and adults (12 years and older) is 5 mg (one tablet) to 15 mg (three tablets) once a day.

Senna extracts are available with many different brand names and as store brands as well. An example of a popular brand of senna is Senakot, which is also available in combination with docusate as Sennakot-S.

– Laxatives may be given as suppositories as well. Liquid glycerin and bisacodyl suppositories are both available over-the-counter and one per day of either may be recommended.

– It is common to give multiple laxatives at the same time though it is not clear how effective that strategy is (Every-Palmer et al., 2017).

Advanced (level 3) measures

If these simpler measures are not sufficient, other interventions may be considered. But, these options either come with the possibility of significant side effects or are expensive or both.

Please note that:

1. No medication is FDA-approved for the treatment of clozapine-induced constipation

2. Out of the medications listed below, the mechanism of action of bethanechol makes it specific for severe constipation caused by a medication with strong anticholinergic properties, like clozapine. But, the

others may be used for constipation of several types, not only for clozapine-induced constipation.

3. Only one of the medications listed below (orlistat) was evaluated in a randomized, clinical trial for the treatment of clozapine-induced constipation. For the others, we only have published case reports.

4. Several of the medications listed below are only available as branded preparations and, so, are quite expensive. Once the branded ones out of these medications become generic, which will happen eventually, we'll have more options for the treatment of constipation.

Anyway, here are some options. They are listed here in no particular order.

— Consider bethanechol (Poetter and Stewart, 2013). Bethanechol is an agonist at muscarinic cholinergic receptors. It was found to be effective in a published case of severe clozapine-induced constipation (Poetter and Stewart, 2013). But, the cholinergic effects of bethanechol can lead to undesirable effects on the gastrointestinal tract (vomiting, abdominal cramping, increased gastric acid secretion), bronchoconstriction, or atrioventricular block (Poetter and Stewart, 2013). Bethanechol is generic and very inexpensive.

— Consider orlistat? Orlistat (brand name Xenical) is a medication that is FDA-approved for weight loss in overweight adults. It acts by decreasing the absorption of fat from the intestine. The increased fat in the stool makes the stool softer and, so, reduces constipation. A double-blind, placebo-controlled clinical trial found that orlistat reduced clozapine-induced constipation (Chukhin et al., 2013). It may seem that orlistat is a great option because it can treat constipation as well as weight gain (Joffe et al., 2008; Tchoukhine et al., 2011), killing two birds with one stone, so to speak. But, the use of orlistat requires that the patient cooperates with taking a low-fat diet, otherwise significant gastrointestinal side effects occur. This is hard for patients with serious mental illness to do. Also, as of March 2020, orlistat is only available as a branded medication and costs about $700 per month!

— Lubiprostone (brand name Amitiza) is a prescription medication (a prostaglandin E1 analog that increases secretions into the intestine) that is FDA-indicated for certain types of constipation. It was found to be effective in a published case of treatment-resistant constipation associated with clozapine (Myers and Cummings, 2014). As of March 2020, lubiprostone is only available as a branded medication and costs about $290 per month (source: goodrx.com).

– Prucalopride (brand name Motegrity), a 5-HT4 receptor agonist, was effective for clozapine-induced constipation in two published cases (Thomas et al., 2018). Prucalopride is FDA-approved for certain types of constipation. Prucalopride is only available as a branded medication and costs about $450 per month (source: goodrx.com).

There are also some other prescription medications whose use in clozapine-induced constipation has not been published as of March 2020, but which may be considered as well:

– Linaclotide (brand name Linzess) is FDA-approved for various types of constipation. It is a guanylate cyclase-C agonist that increases secretion into the intestine and also the motility of the gut. As of March 2020, linaclotide is only available as a branded medication and costs about $460 per month (source: goodrx.com).

– A related medication, plecanatide (brand name Trulance) works by the same mechanism, is also FDA-approved for certain types of constipation, is also available as brand name only, and also costs about $460 per month (source: goodrx.com).

Management of severe constipation

If constipation is severe, the patient should be referred elsewhere for evaluation and management.

If bowel obstruction is ruled out, the treating clinician may recommend measures like manual disimpaction of the stools followed by aggressive treatment of the constipation to prevent a recurrence.

FDA's warning about clozapine-induced constipation

In January 2020, the FDA strengthened an existing warning about clozapine-induced constipation because it noted that:

"Constipation is a frequent and known side effect of clozapine, but serious and fatal events continue to be reported."

From 2006 to 2016, 10 cases of constipation progressing to serious bowel problems resulting in hospitalization, surgery, or death were either reported to the FDA or published in the medical literature. The median time to onset of serious bowel complications was 46 days (range 3 days to 6 months).

The warning and news release discuss some points that we have already covered in this section. Also, it nicely summarizes what we should tell patients, which I am slightly paraphrasing here.

We should ask patients to contact us if:

— The bowel movements are less frequent than normal for them

— They do not have a bowel movement at least three times a week

— They have hard or dry stools

— They have difficulty passing stools, or

— They have difficulty passing gas

Patients should also be told that the situation may be more serious if the patient has any of the following and they should contact a health care professional immediately:

— Nausea/ vomiting

— Abdominal distension

— Abdominal pain

DIARRHEA

Diarrhea associated with mood stabilizers

Many different psychotropic medications can cause diarrhea, including SSRIs, SNRIs, lithium, valproate, etc. About 10% of patients on lithium develop diarrhea (Vestergaard et al., 1988). Among the mood stabilizers, lithium is more likely to cause diarrhea than valproate (Cipriani et al., 2013).

While diarrhea due to mood stabilizers is usually benign, sometimes it can be a sign of toxicity and, in rare cases, of a form of colitis.

Diarrhea is one of the commonest reasons why patients stop taking lithium (Öhlund et al., 2018).

In this section, we'll discuss some simple strategies for managing diarrhea related to the use of mood stabilizers like lithium, valproate, and carbamazepine.

Serum level?

It is not clear to what extent the prevalence of diarrhea increases with higher serum lithium levels. One study found a higher incidence of diarrhea with serum lithium levels greater than 0.8 mEq/L (Vestergaard et al., 1988). But, another paper did not find diarrhea to be related to the dose or serum level (Persson, 1977). But still, diarrhea can be a manifestation of too high a serum level of lithium or valproate. So, we should make sure the serum level is not too high and, if clinically feasible, consider lowering the dose of the medication, at least temporarily.

Reassure the patient

Lithium-induced diarrhea tends to occur in the first 6 months and then tends to subside (Vestergaard et al., 1988). So, we can reassure the patient about this.

This other significance of knowing that diarrhea associated with mood stabilizers tends to occur in the first few months is that if it occurs later on, we should immediately suspect toxicity.

Taking the medication after food?

We all know that to reduce nausea, medications that may cause nausea should be taken after food. But, you may be surprised to know that diarrhea also tends to improve if the lithium or valproate is taken after food (Jeppsson and Sjögren, 1975).

Change to a delayed-release or sustained-release preparation?

I recommend following a general principle that sustained-release preparations tend to have fewer side effects. But, delayed-release or sustained-release preparations are more likely to cause diarrhea than immediate-release preparations (Edström and Persson, 1977). This is probably because the medication is released lower down in the gastrointestinal tract.

LOSS OF APPETITE (ANOREXIA)

Tips to manage loss of appetite due to a stimulant (in adults)

Loss of appetite is a common adverse effect of stimulant medication. It may occur more often in females than in males (Davis et al., 2012). For many adult patients, some weight loss is welcome. However, in some cases, it becomes a concern and must be managed in order to allow the stimulant to continue.

General Measures

1. We can wait and watch because in many cases appetite suppression stabilizes after several weeks.

2. Eat early in the morning before the medication is taken or before it has reached its peak effect. Of course, this can have an effect on the onset of effect of the stimulant, either hastening or delaying the onset.

3. Eat late in the evening after the medication has worn off. This can include a bedtime snack. This has been very effective in my patients.

4. Carry snacks with you everywhere you go. For example, packets of nuts, bananas, cereal bars, etc. Whatever is convenient to carry with you. Eating small amounts throughout the day is easier. It is also good for the ADHD brain, in general, to keep the blood sugar relatively steady through the day.

5. Take one multivitamin/ multimineral pill every day. This will take care of one aspect of this problem by preventing any deficiency of micronutrients.

6. Weigh yourself once a week, in minimal or no clothing, in the morning. (Our weight changes from morning to evening.) Write your weight down and share it with your doctors. Monitoring is key to managing any problem.

7. Eat high-calorie foods whenever possible. For example, among fruits, it is better to eat bananas, pears, mangoes, etc. and to avoid low-calorie fruits like apples, cantaloupe, watermelon.

Medication Changes

1. Consider changing to a shorter-acting preparation. This can allow the medication to wear off between doses and at the end of the day and to allow the appetite to return.

2. Here's a very useful tip: Consider adding mirtazapine (Remeron®) at bedtime. Using a stimulant and mirtazapine (Remeron®) is a GREAT combination for many persons because it can help them sleep better (often a problem) as well as improve their appetite.

3. Similarly, consider adding cyproheptadine (Periactin®). Like mirtazapine (Remeron®), this also stimulates appetite and helps with sleep. However, I usually prefer mirtazapine (Remeron®) over cyproheptadine for my patients because cyproheptadine is antiserotonergic and can counteract the effects of an SSRI if the person is taking one in addition to the stimulant. Cyproheptadine comes in 4 mg strength and the dose can be gradually increased, if needed and tolerated, from 4 mg at bedtime to 16 mg at bedtime.

4. Dose reduction does usually work and may be unavoidable in some cases.

5. There is some data to suggest that amphetamines may produce greater appetite suppression than methylphenidate. If otherwise appropriate, consider switching to methylphenidate as an option in cases of weight loss. This is probably not a high yield option, but I mention is as an option.

6. Changing to a non-stimulant medication for ADHD should be the last resort. After all, there was a good reason that the stimulant was chosen in the first place. Atomoxetine can also cause appetite suppression, but probably less so than the stimulants

NAUSEA

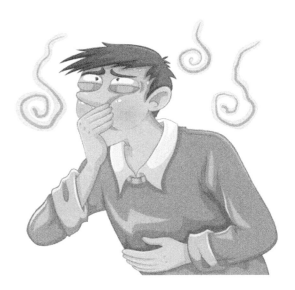

Introduction

Why is medication-induced nausea so important for us to learn to prevent and manage? Nausea is one of the commonest side effects of psychotropic medications and is one of the leading causes of discontinuation of commonly used psychotropic medications. If you have ever had nausea due to any reason, you know that while some other symptoms can be borne, nausea is very difficult to tolerate.

[*Optional to read* (brief philosophical musing): It seems that animals—and, sorry but we are animals too—are biologically programmed to experience nausea and vomiting. This has evolutionary advantages because the potentially poisonous contents of the stomach are ejected from the body. Maybe that is why we find nausea to be a particular unacceptable symptom?]

Please remember! When a patient complains of nausea, we must do something! We shouldn't ask the patient to simply bear with it, because some patients will stop the medication. They may or may not come back to us to ask what to do next.

Think of pancreatitis or drug-induced liver injury

When a patient complains of nausea, vomiting, or abdominal pain, we should think about the possibility of pancreatitis or drug-induced liver injury.

A few characteristics of medication-related nausea that is not medically serious are as follows:

1. Benign nausea due to antidepressant medications develops almost immediately after the patient first starts taking the medication.

2. Also, it is not associated with severe abdominal pain, or other systemic symptoms like fever, jaundice, and so on.

3. And, lastly, it tends to diminish over a week or two.

So, if nausea starts after the patient has been on the medication for a few weeks, if other systemic symptoms are present, and if the nausea gets worse over time instead of better, this suggests that this may not be "benign" nausea. The nausea may be due to liver disease or pancreatitis. If there is any doubt at all that this may be something other than benign medication-induced nausea, we should promptly check hepatic function tests and both serum amylase and serum lipase.

Medication-induced nausea: Level 1 (basic) strategies for prevention and management

Treat pre-existing acid pepsin disease or gastroesophageal reflux disease (GERD) if present

These patients seem to more prone to developing gastrointestinal side effects, including nausea. In such patients, preventive measures should be instituted. For patients with GERD, this may include the use of proton pump inhibitors (PPI). I have treated several such patients successfully by prescribing a PPI before or along with an antidepressant.

In this regard, please remember that omeprazole (but probably NOT other PPIs) increases levels of citalopram and escitalopram.

Reassure the patient

If there is no reason to suspect liver, pancreatic, or other disease as the cause of the nausea, patients should be reassured that the nausea, while distressing, is not "medically dangerous" and that in almost all cases, it diminishes and goes away within a few days or a couple of weeks. It is frustrating for me to see that large numbers of patients have their medications stopped and switched because of transient adverse effects like nausea.

Start at a low dose and titrate up

Sometimes, very simple things that we do clinically can be very helpful. One such thing is asking patients to start the medication at a low dose and then increase later if tolerated.

This doesn't have to be complicated and doesn't have to take a long time. For example, in the case of SSRIs and SNRIs, I typically recommend starting at half of the intended dose. I tell the patient to start by taking half of the intended dose and, if there is no problem, to increase to the intended dose after six or eight days. An even number of days is chosen so as to not waste half a pill. ☐ An example would be to prescribe escitalopram 10 mg tablets but ask the patient to take half a pill for at least four days (more if necessary) and increase

This is not only based on clinical experience. In a specific study of this strategy, when duloxetine was directly started at 60 mg/day, the incidence of nausea was 33% and when it was started at 30 mg/day for one week and then increased to 60 mg/day, the incidence of nausea was 16% (Dunner et al., 2006). 33% vs. 16%. That's a big difference!

Bottom line: Let's ALWAYS start on half of the intended dose.

Take the medication after food

Prevention is better than cure, so any medication that can potentially cause nausea should be given after food.

I used to ask patients to take their SSRI "after breakfast." But, later, I realized that some people have light breakfasts. Or they skip breakfast. Surprisingly, it was not uncommon that this led some patients to take the medication on an empty stomach. So, now I ask patients to take the medication after the first big meal of the day explaining that if they don't eat a significant breakfast, they can take the medication after lunch.

Also, when I told patients to take the medication "with food," some of them thought it was fine to take the medication at the start of the meal. So, now the words I use are "after food."

Switch to a delayed-release or sustained-release preparation

If applicable, switch to a delayed-release or sustained release preparation. Examples of this would be changing from paroxetine to paroxetine controlled-release or divalproex to divalproex extended-release.

Because these preparations release the medication lower down in the GI tract, they may be associated with a lower incidence of nausea. This is not a panacea though; duloxetine, which is a delayed-release preparation, is frequently associated with nausea.

Split the dose

If a patient has nausea from a medication, it may be helpful to split the dose even if the dose does not otherwise need to be split based on the duration of action. This is particularly true for medications that are not sustained-release preparations.

If a patient is taking two medications that cause nausea, tell the patient to take those medications after different meals rather than together after the same meal.

If a patient is prone to nausea or is experiencing nausea, in my clinical experience it often helps to take a spoonful of peanut butter before taking the medication. The peanut butter, having a high fat content, coats the stomach and reduces stomach irritation.

Ask the patient to take ginger in some form

Other than the simple instructions discussed above, the simplest treatment of medication-induced nausea is to ask the patient to take ginger root.

Medication-induced nausea: Level 2 (intermediate) strategies for prevention and management

When the basic (Level 1) strategies don't work, what should we do next?

5-HT3 antagonists

What about the "Setrons," i.e., ondansetron, granisetron, etc.? These medications have been extensively used for the treatment of nausea/vomiting in various medical conditions, including chemotherapy-induced nausea. Nausea associated with SSRIs and SNRIs is believed to be due to excessive stimulation of 5-HT3 receptors and the setrons work by blocking the post-synaptic serotonin-3 (5-HT3) receptors.

Two questions could come up in the readers' minds. Since the setrons block postsynaptic 5-HT3 receptors, could doing this reduce the therapeutic effects of the medications as well? The answer is No, because the therapeutic effects of serotonergic antidepressants are mainly mediated by 5-HT1 receptors. In fact, mirtazapine blocks both 5-HT2 and 5-HT3 receptors but is nevertheless an effective antidepressant.

Keeping in mind that we are prescribing this for nausea, mode of administration is relevant. Ondansetron is available as an orally disintegrating tablet and granisetron as a transdermal patch.

And what about cost? Aren't the setrons very expensive? Not anymore, since they became generic. For example, 30 pills of ondansetron 4 mg orally disintegrating tablets cost about $25 when paying out of pocket.

Warning! Ondansetron is associated with an increased risk of QTc prolongation. It should be avoided with psychotropic medications that also are associated with an increased risk of QTc prolongation and in patients who have other risk factors for QTc prolongation.

Mirtazapine

In addition to its antidepressant and antianxiety effects, mirtazapine has an antinausea effect due to its blockade of 5-HT3 receptors, at which its affinity is similar to that of the "setron" medications (discussed above). Thus, the addition of mirtazapine has been used as a treatment for nausea. Of course, this option for the treatment of nausea would be chosen only if there was another reason for using mirtazapine in that particular patient. But sometimes we can kill two birds with one stone. (Sorry, animal lovers. We need to come up with an alternative proverb!)

Metoclopramide

Metoclopramide is an effective anti-nausea agent. What makes it a great antiemetic is that it works on multiple mechanisms related to nausea. It blocks D2 receptors that mediate nausea at the area postrema in the brainstem and 5-HT3 receptors that mediate nausea caused by serotonergic medications. It moves gastric contents in the right direction by doing three things: it increases the tone (closing) of the lower esophageal sphincter, it decreases the tone of the pyloric sphincter, and it increases peristalsis moving the stomach contents into the small intestine.

Metoclopramide is a prescription medication and is prescribed at 10 mg every 8 hours as needed. While it is true that metoclopramide can occasionally be associated with akathisia (and, rarely, with dystonia), the concern that it may be associated with tardive dyskinesia is not valid because it would only be used for a few days.

PANCREATITIS

Valproate-induced pancreatitis

Here are some key facts about valproate-induced pancreatitis:

– The Prescribing Information for divalproex carries a boxed warning about the risk of pancreatitis.

– It is uncommon but not as rare as is commonly believed (Gerstner et al., 2007).

– It is more common in younger persons but can occur at any age (Asconape et al., 1993)

– The findings can range from asymptomatic elevation of serum amylase to serious disease. Many patients have recovered rapidly once the valproate was stopped. But, rapid progression and several deaths have also been reported.

– It is not clearly associated with the serum level of the medication (Werlin and Fish, 2006; Cofini et al., 2015).

– It can occur either early on or later in the course of treatment (Werlin and Fish, 2006; Cofini et al., 2015).

– But, it is most likely to occur in the first three months and 69% of cases occurred in the first year of treatment with valproic acid (Asconape et al., 1993).

Routine monitoring?

If valproate-induced pancreatitis is more common than we think, should we routinely check serum amylase? I have seen several clinicians do that. One study found that 7% of physicians surveyed routinely monitored serum amylase in persons taking valproate (Asconapé et al., 1993).

But, persons on valproate can have increased serum amylase without having clinical features of pancreatitis (Bale et al., 1982; Asconape et al., 1993).

In one study (Bale et al., 1982), 20% of the patients had an asymptomatic elevation of amylase. Only one patient developed pancreatitis. In all the rest, the amylase returned to normal despite continuing the valproate.

So, a diagnosis of pancreatitis should not be made simply based on elevated amylase if the clinical picture doesn't match (Cofini et al., 2015).

When to suspect valproate-induced pancreatitis

Valproate-induced pancreatitis is more common than we think, especially in younger patients. Those using valproate to treat children and adolescents should be particularly vigilant. If a child on valproate presents with atypical abdominal pain, lethargy, or flu-like syndrome, valproate-induced pancreatitis should be considered (Cofini et al., 2015). Nausea and vomiting are also common.

How is it diagnosed?

– When we suspect valproate-induced pancreatitis, we should remember that serum amylase can sometimes be normal in these cases. Serum lipase is more sensitive for identifying this condition (Werlin and Fish, 2006). So, we should order both serum amylase and lipase.

– Serum amylase or lipase more than three times normal suggest pancreatitis in a person who has clinical symptoms suggestive of pancreatitis.

– Imaging studies (e.g., ultrasound, CT scan, MRI, ERCP) are usually done to confirm the diagnosis.

How is it managed?

– If valproate-induced pancreatitis is suspected, valproate should be stopped immediately.

– The patient should be seen immediately by a primary care physician or gastroenterologist, or sent to the ER for further evaluation and management.

– Rechallenge with valproate is dangerous because the risk of recurrence of pancreatitis is high (Asconape et al., 1993). So, rechallenge should be avoided (Werlin and Fish, 2006; Cofini et al., 2015).

So, it is recommended that if the pancreatitis was thought to be due to the valproate, the patient should NOT be given valproate in the future.

References: See https://simpleandpractical.com/side-effects-references

CHAPTER 10: GENITALS/SEXUALITY

SEXUAL DYSFUNCTION

Antidepressant-induced sexual dysfunction

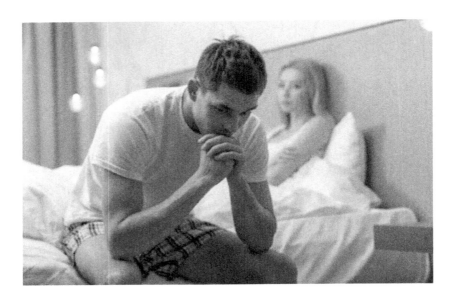

After adverse effects that occur when an antidepressant is first started have subsided, certain longer-term adverse effects persist. The main ones are: sexual dysfunction, weight gain, insomnia, and excessive sweating. These can be very bothersome and which are major causes of non-adherence to antidepressant treatment. Of these longer-term adverse effects of serotonergic antidepressants, sexual dysfunction is particularly frustrating for patients. I have heard several psychiatrists say that their patients don't care too much about the sexual dysfunction but there is considerable data to indicate that patients with depressive disorders do care a lot about this adverse effect, listing it as among the top three adverse effects that they would like to avoid when taking antidepressants. Maybe the patients who cared voted with their feet and are no longer taking the antidepressant or at least no longer seeing the psychiatrist who did not think this adverse effect is a big deal?

Antidepressants can cause problems with different phases of the sexual response cycle: desire, arousal, and orgasm, but especially with orgasm. The incidence of antidepressant-induced sexual dysfunction varies depending on the antidepressant and on the methodology by which the sexual dysfunction was identified. Reviewing the data shows that sexual dysfunction attributable to the antidepressant occurs in about 25% to 50% of patients. That is a lot of people!

Management of antidepressant-induced sexual dysfunction

Important preliminary questions:

1. <u>Are there any other factors that may be entirely or partially causing the sexual dysfunction?</u>

2. <u>Can the antidepressant be stopped?</u>

This is not a silly question. There are many patients in whom the need for antidepressant medication was unclear in the first place. Or, this was a single episode and longer-term maintenance treatment is not required.

Low-yield strategies that work sometimes but not often:

3. <u>Wait and watch</u>

This may be fine to try if the patient is truly willing to try this and understands that you will do more if simply waiting does not work. Unfortunately, antidepressant-induced sexual dysfunction subsides in only 10% of cases. It may show partial improvement in another 10% of patients. If the depression has not yet resolved and/or if this is early in treatment (few weeks or months), it is not unreasonable to decide, collaboratively with the patient, to wait and watch. However, I must strongly emphasize that it is a huge problem that clinicians keep waiting until patients get fed up and stop the medication on their own.

4. <u>Can the dose of the antidepressant be reduced?</u>

Sexual dysfunction is, generally speaking, a dose-dependent adverse effect and can improve if the dose is reduced. This strategy could be particularly useful if in this particular patient the sexual dysfunction only appeared or became significant at a higher dose AND the higher dose was not more helpful for the depression. However, while lowering the dose should certainly be considered as a simple option, it is frequently not a good idea given that it may increase the risk of worsening or relapse.

5. Changing to another serotonergic antidepressant

Changing to another SSRI may be tried, but I must caution that this only works sometimes. Since the sexual dysfunction is directly related to the increased serotonergic activity, the new SSRI is likely to have the same adverse effect.

Strategies that are more promising than the ones above:

6. Drug holidays

The strategy of "drug holidays" for antidepressant-induced sexual dysfunction has been formally tested in only one small, uncontrolled study, but given the limited number of things that have been shown in randomized, controlled trials, it is worth keeping as an option. Some of my patients have obtained meaningful benefit from doing drug holidays.

Now, doing drug holidays is not as simple as you one may think. Which patients or antidepressants could drug holidays be unsuitable for?

a. Antidepressant with a long half-life.

Drug holidays will not work for patients who are on fluoxetine. Why do you think that is? Because has an active metabolite, norfluoxetine, with a long half-life (5 to 7 days).

b. Higher risk of significant discontinuation symptoms.

Drug holidays can be problematic and even dangerous if patients have significant discontinuation symptoms. Therefore, we should ask patients whether they have ever, for any reason, missed this antidepressant for one or more days. If so, did the patient have bothersome discontinuation symptoms?

Discontinuation symptoms are more likely to occur with certain antidepressants. Which ones are these? Paroxetine and venlafaxine are two prominent examples.

In both these cases — long half-life antidepressant and higher risk of discontinuation symptoms — if this is worth the trouble and the potential risk, the patient could be changed to a different antidepressant first before trying the drug holiday.

c. Patients for whom having sexual activity once or twice a week is not sufficient

Such patients are also not suitable for the drug holiday approach as a longer-term solution. However, it may still be of some use in helping the patient continue the antidepressant while other strategies are being considered.

What instructions should be given to the patient regarding drug holidays?

The patient should be asked to miss taking the antidepressant (or to significantly reduce its dose) for two days in a week. Typically, these would be Friday and Saturday mornings. In many cases, this leads to a rapid reduction in the sexual dysfunction and the person is encouraged to attempt to have sex towards the end of this period. If the medication is missed on Friday and Saturday mornings, then the best time to have sex would be on Saturday night or, even better, Sunday morning before taking the morning dose of the antidepressant.

7. Addition of bupropion

While addition of bupropion to an SSRI or SNRI has been recommended for many years as an antidote to antidepressant-induced sexual dysfunction, in the past neither data nor clinical experience has clearly supported its use. Only three randomized, placebo-controlled trials of this strategy have been conducted in the US, and all three were negative (Masand et al., 2001; Clayton et al., 2004; DeBattista et al., 2005).

In the studies cited above, patients were in remission from depression. However, sometimes clinicians add bupropion to an SSRI or SNRI in patients who are not fully in remission. In such cases, a distinction should be made between improvement in the remaining symptoms of depression and improvement in the antidepressant-induced sexual dysfunction per se.

In adding bupropion to an SSRI or SNRI, it should be kept in mind that bupropion is an inhibitor of cytochrome P450 2D6. Therefore, when it is added to duloxetine, fluoxetine, paroxetine, venlafaxine, or vortioxetine, their levels may increase and this may lead to increased adverse effects.

8. Addition of a phosphodiesterase inhibitor

As in patients with erectile dysfunction due to other reasons, phosphodiesterase inhibitors like sildenafil (Viagra) and tadalafil (Cialis) are efficacious in a considerable proportion of patients with antidepressant-induced sexual dysfunction. Tadalafil (Cialis) has a longer duration of action; therefore, it offers greater flexibility regarding the timing of sexual activity. In my opinion, all psychiatrists should familiarize themselves with these tadalafil and prescribe it to their patients when appropriate rather than requiring a consultation with a urologist or primary care physician.

How often does antidepressant-induced sexual dysfunction resolve spontaneously?

Antidepressant-induced sexual dysfunction is very common, distressing to patients, and one of the commonest causes of discontinuation of antidepressants.

Clinicians often reassure patients that it is likely that antidepressant-induced sexual dysfunction, like many side effects, is likely to subside over time. I know because, earlier in my career, I often said this to my patients. This is why wait-and-watch is very commonly recommended by prescribing clinicians. In one large study, the commonest strategy used, by 42% of physicians, was to wait for spontaneous remission of the sexual dysfunction (Bonnierbale et al., 2003).

How often does spontaneous improvement occur?

In two studies from the same group, when patients with antidepressant-induced sexual dysfunction were followed up for six months, the sexual dysfunction resolved in about 10%, partially improved in another 10%, and was unchanged in 80% of patients (Montejo-González et al., 1997; Montejo et al., 2001).

What if the follow up was longer? We don't have great research data on this but in one study with variable follow up, up to three years, "accommodation" to antidepressant-induced sexual dysfunction occurred in only 10% of patients (Ashton and Rosen, 1998).

Bottom line

The problem with overdoing the wait-and-watch approach is that patients get fed up and stop the medication on their own.

It may be OK to wait and watch if:

– It is truly a collaborative decision

– The patient understands that we will do more if simply waiting does not work

– The depression has not yet resolved; that is, further improvement in the depression may improve sexual functioning

– It is early in the treatment, that is, a few weeks or months into the treatment (Zajecka et al., 2001).

– The antidepressant-induced sexual dysfunction is related to orgasm rather than to desire or arousal (Montejo-González et al., 1997).

Trazodone and priapism

Trazodone is a medication that is often used as a hypnotic, especially in persons who are at risk of substance use. However, we know that there is a small risk of priapism associated with it. Here are a few things about trazodone and priapism that we should know:

1. A substantial proportion of persons who develop ischemic priapism permanently lose the ability to have an erection.

2. We should not assume that the risk of priapism is insignificant when a low dose is used as a hypnotic. The risk of priapism doesn't seem to be clearly dose related.

3. Patients may ask how much the risk is. What should we say? The answer: somewhere between 1 in 1000 and 1 in 10,000.

4. Priapism can occur in persons who have been on trazodone for several weeks, especially if there has been an increase in dose.

5. Prolonged erections are often noticed first thing in the morning upon awakening.

Here are THREE things we should do to reduce the risk of priapism and of the potential damage from it. They can be remembered by the mnemonic AIM: *Avoid, Inform, Monitor.*

Before even prescribing trazodone: AVOID

The most practical thing we can do to reduce the risk of priapism with trazodone is to avoid trazodone if possible in certain situations because there is an increased risk of priapism. This is very important. Very serious damage has been reported in persons with these risk factors who were given trazodone.

What are these higher risk situations?

Here are some that many of us encounter commonly:

1) Current or recent cocaine abuse

2) Also taking a PDE-5 inhibitor like sildenafil (Viagra®), tadalafil (Cialis®), vardenafil (Levitra®), etc.

3) Also taking another medication with significant alpha-blocking properties, e.g., risperidone (Risperdal®), prazosin, terazosin, etc.

Less commonly, we may encounter patients with one of these medical conditions and should avoid trazodone in them if possible:

1) Sickle cell anemia or sickle cell trait

2) Leukemia

3) Autonomic dysfunction

4) Hypercoagulable states

Note: This is not a complete risk of clinical situations where the risk of priapism is increased.

While prescribing trazodone: INFORM

It is clear that many patients who develop priapism have delaying treatment because they were initially embarrassed to seek help. This is very unfortunate because the key to reducing the chances of serious damage to the penis resulting from the priapism is to treat it as early as possible.

Therefore, if there is one thing we must tell male patients to whom we prescribe trazodone, it is that in rare cases they could develop persistent painful erections and if this happens they should not wait and MUST go to the emergency room WITHOUT DELAY because serious damage to the penis can occur. We must also document that we told the patient this.

After prescribing trazodone: MONITOR

Another sad thing is that in up to 50% of men who subsequently developed priapism, it was preceded by prolonged erections. So many of the cases of priapism could have been prevented if the person had been asked about the presence of prolonged erections and, if it was present, the trazodone had been stopped.

Therefore, when seeing men who are taking trazodone, we must ask about any prolonged erections and immediately stop the trazodone if prolonged erections are occurring.

Arizona Sexual Experiences Scale (ASEX)

The Arizona Sexual Experiences Scale (ASEX) is a questionnaire commonly used in clinical trials to assess sexual functioning.

The Scale

The ASEX has 5 questions pertaining to different aspects of sexual functioning. These are:

1. Desire: "How strong is your sex drive?"
2. Arousal: "How easily are you sexually aroused (turned on)?"
3. Penile erection or vaginal lubrication: "Can you easily get and keep an erection?" or "How easily does your vagina become moist or wet during sex?"
4. Orgasm: "How easily can you reach an orgasm?"

5.   Satisfaction: "Are your orgasms satisfying?"

Each item is scored from 1 to 6 with each score having a brief, simple anchor.

For example, the first item has the following anchor points for scoring: 1 "extremely strong," 2 "very strong," 3 "somewhat strong," 4 "somewhat weak," 5 "very weak," 6 "no sex drive."

Item 2 has the following anchor points: 1 "extremely easily," 2 "very easily," 3 "somewhat easily," 4 "somewhat difficult," 5 "very difficult," 6 "never aroused."

The instructions simply state: "For each item, please indicate your OVERALL level during the PAST WEEK, including TODAY."

Administration and Scoring

The advantage of the ASEX is that it is simple to administer and easy to score. It can be completed by the subject on his or her own, or the questions can be asked by the clinician.

Since there are 5 questions and each is scored from 1 to 6, the total score is from 5 to 30. Notice that it is not from zero to 30.

Sexual dysfunction is defined as:

Total 19 or more, OR

5 or more on any item, OR

4 or more on three items

Dr. Cynthia McGahuey, the first author for this scale, reminds us that low scores represent normal sexual function and high scores represent the presence of sexual dysfunction (personal communication). A few articles have incorrectly stated the opposite about the ASEX scale in terms of what the scores mean.

She pointed out that extremely low scores could also represent sexual dysfunction (i.e., hyperfunction), examples of which are premature ejaculation or spontaneous orgasm.

Importantly, she asks us to remember that the ASEX was designed to determine whether sexual dysfunction was present and to what degree, not the etiology of it.

The ASEX scale has been translated into over a dozen languages other than English.

Note: The scale is copyrighted by the Arizona Board of Regents and all rights are reserved by them.

An introduction to the Changes in Sexual Functioning Questionnaire (CSFQ)

The problem

Sexual functioning is a sensitive topic, even among patients in Western countries. It has been shown that patients are reluctant to spontaneously report problems with sexual functioning, either as a medication side effect or due to other reasons.

What is a possible solution to the under-reporting of problems with sexual functioning?

It is also known that patients frequently stop taking their medication because they believe it is affecting their sexual functioning, whether that is the case or not.

If sexual functioning is systematically assessed and documented even before a medication is started, this can be extremely helpful in monitoring any change after the medication is started.

The solution

The solution is to use a questionnaire that patients can fill out outside of the clinical session on their own time. This has three advantages:

1. It has been shown that people are much more open about difficulties with sexual functioning when asked by a self-report questionnaire than they are when asked by an interviewer.

2. It does not take up any time during the clinical visit where we are already short of time.

3. It may introduce the topic of sexual functioning to the patient.

Which questionnaire should we use?

The questionnaire should not be so brief that it doesn't get any details of functioning in the different phases of the sexual cycle. But it should also not be so long that patients are reluctant to complete the questionnaire.

The Changes in Sexual Functioning Questionnaire (CSFQ) is a well-established questionnaire that has been extensively validated. It has been used in dozens of clinical trials of psychotropic medications.

The 14-item version is the version recommended for clinical use. It only takes three to five minutes for the patient to complete the questionnaire.

There are a Male and a Female versions of the questionnaire. The questions about desire and pleasure are the same for men and women. But, of course, the questions about arousal and orgasm are different for men and women.

The CSFQ has been validated in the US and in Spain (in Spanish). It has been translated into at least 75 languages!

Copyright issues

The CSFQ is copyrighted by Anita H. Clayton, MD who is also on the Editorial Board of Simple and Practical Mental Health.

There is a fee for use of the CSFQ in commercially-sponsored research.

For permission to use the scale in research with other types of funding or no funding, please contact Dr. Clayton.

How to administer, score, and interpret the Changes in Sexual Functioning Questionnaire (CSFQ)

Important instructions while giving the CSFQ to the patient

1. It is important that subjects read the introductory paragraph explaining what types of sexual behavior/activity are referred to in the scale. Otherwise, they may wrongly think that the questionnaire is only asking about sex with another person.

The introductory paragraph states:

"NOTE: This is a questionnaire about sexual activity and sexual function. By sexual activity, we mean sexual intercourse, masturbation, sexual fantasies and other activity."

2. An instruction that is not noted on the questionnaire but I recommend we explicitly tell each patient each time we give any patient-rated questionnaire is to make sure that every question is answered. It is quite common for patients to skip one or more questions by mistake. This becomes a headache in terms of interpretation of the total score. Dr. Clayton has provided some guidelines for what to do if one or more questions are skipped but they are not discussed in this section.

3. Time-frame for answering the questions

The questionnaire itself does not include this instruction, so we need to tell the patient that:

– The first time the CSFQ is administered, the questions should be answered in relation to the previous one month

– After that, usually we ask patients to answer the questions with regard to sexual activity since the last time the CSFQ was done. But, if appropriate, we can modify this instruction.

So, let's say a patient makes an appointment for an initial evaluation. In the paperwork to be completed before we see the patient, we provide a copy of the CSFQ and ask the patient to answer it with regard to the previous one month. If a medication is started and the patient comes back in two weeks, it may be appropriate to ask the patient to do the questionnaire with regard to the previous two weeks since starting the medication. Now, let's say it is three months since the medication was started. Then, we may prefer to ask the patient to answer the questions in relation to the previous two or four weeks in order to understand the current sexual functioning. e.g., improvement with treatment of the condition.

How to score the CSFQ

So, you gave or sent the Changes in Sexual Functioning Questionnaire to your patient along with the instructions as discussed in the last two emails. The patient gives you back the filled out questionnaire. The next step is to score it.

Immediately check to make sure that all questions on the questionnaire have been answered.

The score on each item is the numerical score of the answer chosen by the patient.

For example, as shown in the image below, in Item 1, a response of "some enjoyment or pleasure" has a numerical value of 3, whereas a response of "much enjoyment or pleasure" has a numerical value of 4.

1. Compared with the most enjoyable it has ever been, how enjoyable or pleasurable is your sexual life right now?
☐ 1-No enjoyment or pleasure
☐ 2-Little enjoyment or pleasure
☐ 3-Some enjoyment or pleasure
☐ 4-Much enjoyment or pleasure
☐ 5-Great enjoyment or pleasure

Note: Items 10 and 14 are reverse-scored. For example, as shown in the image below, on Item 10, a response of "never" has a numerical value of 5, whereas a response of "every day" has a value of 1.

10. How often do you experience painful, prolonged erections?
☐ 5-Never
☐ 4-Rarely (once a month or less)
☐ 3-Sometimes (more than once a month, up to twice a week)
☐ 2-Often (more than twice a week)
☐ 1-Every day

If two answers are marked for one item on the CSFQ AND they are adjacent in value (e.g., a score of 1 and 2 or of 3 and 4), the scores for the two answer choices can be averaged. For example, if on a particular item, both 1 and 2 are chosen by the patient, we can consider the score on that item to be 1.5.

To score the CSFQ, all we have to do is to follow the scoring aid at the bottom of the questionnaire that is shown in the image below.

_____ = Pleasure (Item 1)
_____ = Desire/Frequency (Item 2 + Item 3)
_____ = Desire/Interest (Item 4 + Item 5 + Item 6)
_____ = Arousal/Erection (Item 7 + Item 8 + Item 9)
_____ = Orgasm/Ejaculation (Item 11 + Item 12 + Item 13)
_____ = **Total CSFQ Score** (Items 1 to 14)

In the scoring aid, enter the total of the score on the item or items for each subscale. This gives us five subscale scores.

Note: Items 10 & 14 are not included in the subscale scores, but they are included in the total CSFQ score.

Now, add up all the subscales as shown in the scoring aid to get the Total CSFQ score.

How to interpret CSFQ total and subscale scores

Both the total and subscale scores are important. The CSFQ scores (total and each subscale) that indicate sexual dysfunction are as follows.

Men

Total score 47 or less

Pleasure subscale 4 or less

Desire/frequency subscale 8 or less

Desire/interest subscale 11 or less

Arousal/excitement subscale 13 or less

Orgasm/completion subscale 13 or less

Women

Total score 41 or less

Pleasure subscale 4 or less

Desire/frequency subscale 6 or less

Desire/interest subscale 9 or less

Arousal/excitement subscale 12 or less

Orgasm/completion subscale 11 or less

Which laboratory tests in men with erectile dysfunction?

When a male patient presents with erectile dysfunction that may be due to a psychotropic medication, what lab tests should we order (in addition to tests for general evaluation of the patient's health)?

1. Free testosterone

Low testosterone is present in only about 5% of men with erectile dysfunction (Buvat and Lemaire, 1997). Also, there can be some variability in testosterone levels. So, there is some controversy about whether or not serum testosterone should be checked in all men with erectile dysfunction.

In my opinion, it is worth ordering "serum free and total testosterone" because if testosterone levels are low, treatment with testosterone can significantly improve the sexual dysfunction (Jain et al., 2000).

Also, in men with low-normal testosterone levels, the addition of transdermal testosterone may improve the response to treatment of erectile dysfunction with a PDE5 inhibitor (Alhathal et al., 2012).

If we order serum testosterone and find it to be low, we should refer the patient to a primary care physician or an endocrinologist for further evaluation of the cause of the low testosterone and for possible treatment with testosterone.

2. Serum prolactin

Serum prolactin elevation is found only rarely in men with erectile dysfunction.

BUT, elevated prolactin is an important cause of erectile dysfunction in men receiving potent D2 blocking medications like risperidone or haloperidol.

And, prolactin can be elevated by antidepressants as well.

So, mental health clinicians should consider measuring serum prolactin in men with erectile dysfunction who are on either an antipsychotic or an antidepressant.

How to reduce the risk of erectile dysfunction

If mental health clinicians assess sexual functioning as part of our assessments, as we should, we find that a lot of our male patients have erectile dysfunction. They may be on medications that may cause erectile dysfunction. But, the erectile dysfunction may also be related to our patients tending to be overweight, to smoke, to have cardiovascular disease, etc.

Let's encourage our patients, as early in life as possible, to make lifestyle changes that have been shown to reduce the risk of erectile dysfunction.

1. Weight loss (if overweight/obese)

2. Smoking cessation

3. Regular aerobic exercise

4. Avoiding excessive alcohol

5. Effective control of diabetes/ hypertension/ hyperlipidemia (if applicable).

This point is important for several reasons. As one paper noted:

"Reducing the risk of erectile dysfunction may be a useful and to this point unexploited motivation for men to engage in health-promoting behaviors."

Associations shown in long-term prospective studies

In a prospective, 14-year follow up study of men who did NOT have erectile dysfunction at baseline (Bacon et al., 2006):

– Obesity doubled the risk of developing erectile dysfunction

– Smoking increased the risk by 50% (also see Cao et al., 2013), and

– Engaging in physical exercise reduced the risk by 30%.

It is not clear why weight loss affects erectile dysfunction. It is possible that this may be due to some or several of the following factors (Glina et al., 2013): decreased inflammation, increased serum testosterone levels, improved mood, and improved self-esteem.

But, will making lifestyle changes reduce the risk of developing erectile dysfunction? If so, what exactly should we recommend? Let's discuss these questions next.

Make lifestyle changes earlier in life

These lifestyle changes should be made as early in life as possible. One prospective follow up study found that while obesity, smoking, and lack of exercise were related to the risk of subsequently developing erectile dysfunction, subsequently losing weight or stopping smoking did not clearly reduce the risk of developing erectile dysfunction (Derby et al., 2000).

While this study was not large enough for us to be sure of this, the authors warned that, "Midlife changes may be too late to reverse the effects of smoking, obesity, and alcohol consumption on erectile dysfunction."

But, the good news is that physical exercise, even if started in midlife, did reduce the risk of developing erectile dysfunction.

Also, I wonder if even later in life making the other lifestyle changes might at least reduce further progression of the erectile dysfunction or even reduce its severity.

How much exercise?

To improve already existing erectile dysfunction that is believed to be related to physical inactivity, obesity, hypertension, metabolic syndrome, and/or cardiovascular disease, studies have found that the following level of aerobic exercise helps reduce erectile dysfunction (Gerbild et al., 2018):

– 40 minutes per day

– Moderate to vigorous intensity

– Four (or more) times per week.

This is similar to what is good for general health anyway.

Which PDE-5 inhibitor for erectile dysfunction?

A substance called cyclic GMP, when released, dilates the blood vessels in the penis, which leads to an erection. Cyclic GMP is broken down by an enzyme called phosphodiesterase type 5 (PDE-5). This is why medications that inhibit PDE-5 increase the effect of cyclic GMP and increase penile erections.

These medications are first-line treatments for erectile dysfunction. They have also been shown to effective for antidepressant-induced erectile dysfunction.

Mental health clinicians may recommend a PDE-5 inhibitor for medication-induced sexual dysfunction. We may either prescribe it ourselves or refer the patient to the primary care physician for this. Either way, we should know how to choose between the different PDE-5 inhibitors. Also, one of them should be avoided with medications that may prolong the QT interval.

Let's compare them on:

– Duration of action
– Effect of food
– Onset of action
– Cost
– Risk of additive QT prolongation
– Risk of serious visual disturbance, and
– Other side effects.

Based on these factors, is there one PDE-5 inhibitor that may be considered the best choice?

Available PDE-5 inhibitors

There are four PDE-5 inhibitors available in the US as of May 2018. I made the mnemonic V.A.S.T. to remember their generic names.

Vardenafil (brand name Levitra)

Avanafil (brand name Stendra)

Sildenafil (brand name Viagra)

Tadalafil (brand name Cialis)

Duration of action

The half-life of three of the PDE-5 inhibitors is about 4 to 5 hours.

But for tadalafil, the half-life is about 18 hours. So, the effect of tadalafil lasts for 24 to 36 hours.

This is a big advantage because it means that sexual activity does not need to be timed within a narrow window of opportunity.

Effect of food

High-fat meals significantly increase the time to peak levels and reduce the peak levels for avanafil, sildenafil, and vardenafil. So, the effect of these PDE-5 inhibitors may be both delayed and reduced if the person recently

ate a meal with high-fat content (Rew and Heidelbaugh, 2016).
But the absorption of tadalafil is NOT affected by food.

This is an important advantage in terms of convenience and not needing to time sexual activity in relation to a meal.

Onset of action

The minimum time that the medication takes to work is as follows:

Vardenafil 60 minutes

Avanafil 15 minutes

Sildenafil 30 minutes

Tadalafil 30 minutes

Cost

(updated July 2020)

On goodrx.com in July 2020 for five of the highest strength tablets available:

Vardenafil (brand name Levitra): $64 for five 20 mg tablets

Avanafil (brand name Stendra): $267 for five 200 mg tablets

Sildenafil (brand name Viagra): $11 for five 100 mg tablets

Tadalafil (brand name Cialis): $10 for five 20 mg tablets.

So, sildenafil and tadalafil are the most economical as of July 2020.

Next, let's look at the risk of two serious adverse effects that can occur with the PDE-5 inhibitors.

QT prolongation

Since some psychotropic medications can prolong the QTc interval, the fact that one of the four PDE-5 inhibitors can prolong the QT interval is very relevant to us.

From the Prescribing Information for vardenafil (brand name Levitra; emphasis added by SPMH):

"In a study of the effect of LEVITRA on QT interval in 59 healthy males, therapeutic (10 mg) and supratherapeutic (80 mg) doses of vardenafil and the active control moxifloxacin (400 mg) produced similar increases in QTc interval.

A postmarketing study evaluating the effect of combining LEVITRA with another drug of comparable QT effect showed an additive QT effect when compared with either drug alone.

These observations should be considered in clinical decisions when prescribing LEVITRA to patients with known history of QT prolongation or patients who are taking medications known to prolong the QT interval."

So, we may avoid vardenafil in persons taking a medication that may prolong the QTc interval.

Serious visual disturbance

The PDE-5 inhibitors can, in rare cases, lead to sudden loss of vision in one or both eyes. This is due to inhibition of another PDE subtype (PDE-6) in the retina and is called non-arteritic anterior ischemic optic neuropathy (NAION).

Tadalafil and vardenafil have low affinity for this retinal PDE-6. So, it is possible that their risk of causing NAION may be lower than that for sildenafil (Brock et al., 2002; Mikhail, 2005).

Other side effects

The other side effects of the PDE-5 inhibitors are generally similar for each of them with some exceptions. For example:

– Tadalafil is more than four times as likely as sildenafil to cause myalgia/back pain (Gong et al., 2017).

– Sildenafil is more than twice as likely as tadalafil to cause flushing.

If these side effects occur and are very troublesome, we can try to switch to a different PDE-5 inhibitor, but I don't think these differences affect our initial choice of the PDE-5 inhibitor.

Bottom line

The way I see it, tadalafil (brand name Cialis) is a good choice among the PDE-5 inhibitors due to the longer duration of action, lack of effect of food, lack of QT prolongation, and possibly lower risk of serious eye problems. It seems to have all the advantages.

Beta blockers can worsen or improve erectile dysfunction

Persons with mental health problems often have erectile dysfunction either due to the disorder themselves or due to medications used to the disorders, e.g., antidepressants, antipsychotics.

But, erectile dysfunction in our patients can be multifactorial and/or due to other causes. One such set of causes is some, but not all, antihypertensive medications.

Among the antihypertensives, beta-blockers are associated with an increased risk of erectile dysfunction (Baumhäkel et al., 2011). Mental health clinicians need to know about this both because:

– We sometimes prescribe beta blockers for somatic symptoms of anxiety, tremors, akathisia, etc.

– Many of our patients have hypertension or other cardiovascular disease and may be on a beta-blocker for that

– Erectile dysfunction due to psychotropic medications is common but the erectile dysfunction in our patients may in part be due to other medications like beta-blockers.

The good news is that not all beta-blockers are equally problematic in regard to the risk of erectile dysfunction.

Here is a quick summary of some key things to know in regard to beta-blockers and erectile dysfunction:

– Beta-blockers like propranolol (brand name Inderal) are strongly associated with erectile dysfunction.

– Some newer beta-blockers like carvedilol (brand name Coreg) and celiprolol (not available in the US as of July 2018) may be much less likely to cause erectile dysfunction.

– Nebivolol (brand name Bystolic) also appears to be associated with a lower risk of erectile dysfunction than other beta-blockers (Cordero et al., 2010; Aldemir et al., 2016; Gür et al., 2017).

– Nebivolol, rather than causing erectile dysfunction, may even be associated with improvement in erectile dysfunction (Manolis and Doumas, 2012). What could be a possible mechanism for this? Nebivolol is the only beta-blocker known to potentiate the effects of nitric oxide (Gupta and Wright, 2008). Among other places, nitric oxide is released in the penis during sexual stimulation and leads to the vasodilation that is involved in penile erection. Remember that PDE-5 inhibitors like sildenafil, tadalafil, etc., also work by potentiating the effects of nitric oxide.

What should we do?

1. In every patient with erectile dysfunction, we should look to see what psychotropic and non-psychotropic medications the person is on. These should include beta-blockers.

2. If the person is on a beta-blocker, e.g., for the treatment of hypertension, etc., and has erectile dysfunction we may recommend to the treating clinician (e.g., primary care physician) that a change to nebivolol should be considered.

While this is good news for patients taking a beta-blocker for hypertension, there are a few important questions about nebivolol that we have to think about:

– Could switching from another beta-blocker for the treatment of hypertension to nebivolol worsen the hypertension?

– Is cost a barrier?

– Will some psychotropic medications have a clinically-significant drug interaction with nebivolol?

– In addition to hypertension, can nebivolol also be used for the treatment of medication-induced tremor and/or akathisia?

Let's answer these questions next.

1. Will this change be a poor choice with regard to the treatment of hypertension?

No. In fact, nebivolol is considered to be a good choice for the treatment of hypertension. This is because, along with carvedilol, labetalol, and celiprolol (not available in the US as of July 2018), it has vasodilating effects. These beta-blockers, called third-generation beta-blockers, are preferred in patients with hypertension because they also decrease peripheral vascular resistance.

2. Is cost a barrier?

It can be because nebivolol is not yet available as a cheaper generic. That is expected to happen in the US in 2021.

3. Potential drug interactions with psychotropic medications?

Of relevance to psychopharmacologists, nebivolol is metabolized by cytochrome P450 2D6. In 2D6 poor metabolizers or in those who are also taking a potent 2D6 inhibitor (e.g., fluoxetine, paroxetine), nebivolol loses its beta-1 selectivity and becomes a non-selective beta-blocker, which can lead to increased adverse effects.

4. Can nebivolol also be used for the treatment of medication-induced tremor or akathisia?

– For tremors, yes. While as of July 2018, I am not aware of any published report of using nebivolol for the treatment of tremor, beta-1 selective ("cardioselective") beta blockers that do not cross the blood-brain barrier (because they are lipophilic) do work for tremors and should probably be preferred due to fewer side effects.

– But, nebivolol is not appropriate for the treatment of akathisia. A central effect and non-selective beta blockade seem to be required for an anti-akathisia effect (Miller and Fleischhacker, 2000).

Cyproheptadine (Periactin®) for antidepressant-induced sexual dysfunction (ADISD)?

While antidepressant-induced erectile dysfunction (ADISD) can be treated with PDE-5 inhibitors like sildenafil, tadalafil, etc., but decreased libido, delayed or absent ejaculation in men, and anorgasmia in women are harder to treat.

In this section, we will discuss the potential use of cyproheptadine (brand name Periactin) as a potential treatment for these sexual adverse effects of serotonergic antidepressants.

What is cyproheptadine?

It is a medication that blocks 5-HT2 receptors, histamine-1 receptors, muscarinic cholinergic receptors, and L-calcium channels.

Its FDA indications are for the treatment of several allergic conditions but it has been used off-label in mental health to promote appetite and to treat serotonin syndrome, akathisia, and antidepressant-induced sexual dysfunction (ADISD) even without strong research evidence for these uses.

Why consider cyproheptadine for ADISD?

The sexual dysfunction related to use of serotonergic antidepressants is believed to be related to increased activity at 5-HT2A receptors. This is why antidepressants like mirtazapine, nefazodone, and trazodone that block 5-HT2A receptors are less likely to lead to sexual dysfunction.

How to use cyproheptadine for ADISD

This use of cyproheptadine has not yet been studied in a clinical trial. But, several case reports and case series have reported that cyproheptadine can reverse sexual dysfunction caused by serotonergic antidepressants. When it works, it may allow patients to have an orgasm, which is a great relief to the patients.

I occasionally use cyproheptadine in my patients when other options for treating antidepressant-induced sexual dysfunction are not feasible. Here are some details about how exactly to use cyproheptadine for ADISD:

1. Antidepressant-induced delayed ejaculation in men and anorgasmia in women are the problems for which cyproheptadine is most likely to be used.

2. Delayed ejaculation and anorgasmia are dose-related and the benefit of cyproheptadine is dose-related as well (Lauerma, 1996; Arnott and Nutt, 1994). So, in general, the higher the dose of the serotonergic antidepressant, the higher the dose of cyproheptadine that the patient is likely to need.

3. The dose used typically ranges from 2 mg to 16 mg. I typically start with 4 mg and then go up or down as needed.

4. It is available as a 4 mg tablet, is generic, and inexpensive.

5. Cyproheptadine can be used on an as-needed basis and is typically taken 30 to 60 minutes (or sometimes even two hours) before sexual activity (e.g., Javanbakht, 2015). Patients really like this ability to take the medication only when needed.

6. The patient should be warned about the possible sedation that may persist till the following morning.

7. There have been reports of the reversal of the antidepressant effect (e.g., Feder, 1991; Goldbloom and Kennedy, 1991). Cyproheptadine, like other H-1 antagonists, can also cause weight gain. This is why I recommend that if cyproheptadine is used to treat antidepressant-induced sexual dysfunction, it should only be used on an as-needed basis.

8. I strongly advise the patient to "do a practice run," that is, to try taking the medication before masturbation rather than trying it for the first time when having sex with a partner. If the patient is not willing to do that (very rare in my patients), then the patient should just try it on a day when s/he is not going to have sex. By doing this, patients can get a sense of how helpful and how sedating the medication is going to be for them.

Does bupropion treat antidepressant-induced sexual dysfunction?

Antidepressant-induced sexual dysfunction is:

- Common

- Very bothersome to many patients

- A leading cause of discontinuation of antidepressant treatment by patients

- Unlikely to resolve unless something is done.

A survey of psychiatrists showed that the most common treatment or antidote prescribed to try to reverse sexual dysfunction caused by antidepressants was bupropion—by 43% of the psychiatrists surveyed (Dording et al., 2002). In the past, I too prescribed bupropion for this purpose to many patients with antidepressant-induced sexual dysfunction.

Does it work?

There are five published randomized, placebo-controlled trials that evaluated the use of bupropion as a treatment for antidepressant-induced sexual dysfunction (Masand et al., 2001; Clayton et al., 2004; DeBattista et al., 2005, Safarinejad, 2010; Safarinejad, 2011).

Shouldn't this be a settled question then? Why does controversy persist?

Two of the five studies (Masand et al., 2001; DeBattista et al., 2005): Clear-cut results; zero benefits from adding bupropion.

Another one of these five studies (Clayton et al., 2004) is often quoted as having been "positive," that is, as having shown that bupropion does work for antidepressant-induced sexual dysfunction. I hear this ALL the time! The Conclusion in the Abstract for that paper (yellow highlight added by me) said that it worked:

> **Conclusions:** Bupropion SR, as an effective antidote to SSRI-induced sexual dysfunction, produced an increase in desire to engage in sexual activity and frequency of engaging in sexual activity compared with placebo. A larger study is needed to further investigate this finding.
> *(J Clin Psychiatry 2004;65:62–67)*

Why do I not accept this? I will explain that below.

The main outcome measure in this study was the patient-rated questionnaire called the Changes in Sexual Functioning Questionnaire (CSFQ).

The CSFQ has 14 questions and the answers to these questions are added up as per the directions to give us six numbers: a total score and five subscale scores.

The five subscales are:

1. Pleasure

2. Desire/interest

3. Desire/frequency

4. Arousal/erection

5. Orgasm/ejaculation.

Now, let's see what the Clayton et al. (2004) found regarding the effect of treatment with bupropion on these six numbers:

Total score: No difference

1. Pleasure: Not reported

2. Desire/interest: No difference

3. Desire/frequency: Bupropion > Placebo (p< 0.024)

4. Arousal/erection: No difference

5. Orgasm/ejaculation: No difference

So, sexual interest, erection or arousal, orgasm or ejaculation—none of them improved statistically significantly more than with placebo.

The ONLY thing that improved statistically significantly more in the bupropion group was the desire/frequency subscale. This subscale score is a combination of the score on two questions:

1. How frequently do you engage in sexual activity (sexual intercourse, masturbation, etc.) now?

2. How often do you desire to engage in sexual activity?

So, bupropion improved desire to engage in sexual activity but not sexual desire per se or the ability to engage in and enjoy sex? Maybe in this situation, the patients would be better off with a decreased desire to engage in sexual activity?

Also, if we understand the basic concept of statistical significance, we will realize that the $P < 0.05$ cut off for statistical significance becomes problematic if multiple statistical tests are done.

In that study, there were at several major comparisons made, most importantly, comparing bupropion and placebo on the total CSFQ score and four CSFQ subscales. None of these was pre-specified as a "primary" outcome measure. (If a primary outcome measure had been chosen, I would think it should have been the Total CSFQ score.)

Also, no correction was made to account for the multiple statistical comparisons done. If we correct for even the five main statistical tests (comparisons on the total score and four of the subscales), even the desire/frequency subscale on which the P-value was 0.024 for the comparison between bupropion and placebo would not show a statistically significant benefit for bupropion because only a P-value of 0.05 divided by five or < 0.01 would be considered statistically significant.

If the paragraph above was confusing to you, you can safely ignore it. It won't alter our final conclusion.

Now, until 2010, I lectured on this topic and there was no problem. I would say that three placebo-controlled studies have shown that bupropion is no better than placebo (except for the one isolated area of possible improvement in one study).

What was surprising about these papers from Iran was not only that the findings contradicted the three studies done in the US, but also that only ONE person was the sole author (very unusual) and he claimed to have enrolled and treated very large numbers of patients—sample sizes that were massive compared to all other clinical trials on this topic that were ever done anywhere in the world. But, what could I do? I couldn't say in my lectures that I don't believe the findings of these papers. Why not, I would be asked. On what basis? But, these two papers caused a lot of confusion and uncertainty in the medical literature and among clinicians.

Then, in 2015, the Editor and Publisher of the journal that had published one of the papers officially retracted the paper (Saferinejad, 2015). Here is the Retraction Notice:

Retraction Notice

Retraction statement: The effects of the adjunctive bupropion on male sexual dysfunction induced by a selective serotonin reuptake inhibitor: a double-blind placebo-controlled and randomized study

Retraction: Safarinejad MR (2010), The effects of the adjunctive bupropion on male sexual dysfunction induced by a selective serotonin reuptake inhibitor: a double-blind placebo-controlled and randomized study. *BJU International* 106: 6: 840–7.

The above article, published online on 8th Jan 2010 in Wiley Online Library (wileyonlinelibrary.com), has been retracted by agreement between the journal Editor in Chief, Professor Prokar Dasgupta and John Wiley & Sons Ltd. The retraction has been agreed after an independent review found a pattern of inappropriate statistical analysis.

The other paper has not been retracted but now I feel comfortable saying to you that I think it too should be ignored.

Bottom line

There have three—and only three—credible, randomized, placebo-controlled clinical trials on the use of bupropion for the treatment of antidepressant-induced sexual dysfunction and all three were negative. That is, bupropion is not effective, in general, for antidepressant-induced sexual dysfunction.

But, bupropion may still have a role in these patients if:

– The patient is still depressed

– The problem is mainly one of desire.

References: See https://simpleandpractical.com/side-effects-references

CHAPTER 11: HYPERGLYCEMIA

How long does antipsychotic-induced hyperglycemia take to resolve?

After cross tapering between atypical antipsychotics, how long will it take glucose levels to decrease if they are going to do so?

This is a very clinically relevant question! But like many of the questions I get, not easy to answer.

In this case, the difficulty is because:

– Whether and after how long antipsychotic-induced hyperglycemia improves can be quite variable, and

– The published literature on the subject is quite limited (as of May 2020).

Two DIFFERENT scenarios

The literature is usually not clear about this but antipsychotic-induced hyperglycemia or diabetes can be of two different types:

1. In the majority of cases, the person gains weight, then develops insulin resistance, and, finally, type II diabetes becomes established. In these cases, just like in other cases of type II diabetes, reversing the illness can take a long time. Among other things, the person has to lose a substantial amount of weight before the hyperglycemia improves.

2. In some other cases, the person develops severe hyperglycemia and even diabetic ketoacidosis. This can occur even without significant weight gain. And, it can occur very early in treatment.

Let's look at some published case reports of this type of antipsychotic-induced severe hyperglycemia and see how long it took to resolve after the antipsychotic was stopped or changed. Here are just a few examples:

Case report

A middle-aged obese female who was being treated with quetiapine for two years developed very serious diabetic ketoacidosis (Dibben et al., 2005). Among other things, she was treated with insulin and her quetiapine was stopped. Over the next few months, her insulin requirements progressively dropped and by six months after the episode, her blood sugar was normal even without any medication.

Case report

A young woman who had significant weight gain on clozapine and, after six months on clozapine, had an episode of diabetic ketoacidosis (Strassnig et al., 2013; Case 1). Fasting glucose was 661 mg/dL and hyperlipidemia was present as well. She was treated with insulin and oral hypoglycemics.

Later, due to non-adherence, clozapine was stopped and she was put on a depot injection of a first-generation antipsychotic. Within two weeks after stopping clozapine, her blood sugar was normal without insulin or oral hypoglycemic. Over two years of follow up, her blood sugar and lipids remained normal.

Case report

A middle-aged obese woman in a psychotic relapse was put on olanzapine 30 mg/day (not a great choice!) and risperidone long-acting injection (Strassnig et al., 2013; Case 2). Two weeks later, her blood sugar was 540 mg/dL. She was treated with insulin and maximum doses of oral hypoglycemics. Olanzapine and risperidone were stopped and she was put on a first-generation antipsychotic.

"Within weeks" after making the change, her blood sugar and lipids were normal even without any antidiabetes treatment and remained normal at follow up six months later.

Case report

A middle-aged woman of normal weight was started on clozapine (Strassnig et al., 2013; Case 3). Four weeks later, fasting blood sugar was 144 mg/dL. Despite starting an oral hypoglycemic and though she had not gained weight on the clozapine, the blood glucose worsened over the next few weeks and she also developed hyperlipidemia.

So, the patient was switched to an oral first-generation antipsychotic. In less than two months, the blood sugar returned to normal even though the oral hypoglycemic was stopped. Two months after the diabetes was first diagnosed, her blood sugar was normal.

Bottom line

Second-generation antipsychotics can be associated with either gradual onset of weight gain/ hyperglycemia/ insulin resistance/ type II diabetes or with acute onset of hyperglycemia that may be severe and may lead to diabetic ketoacidosis. Both animal and human studies have shown that antipsychotics like clozapine and olanzapine can lead to impaired insulin sensitivity that can occur quickly (even after a single dose!) and be independent of weight gain (Cohen and Correll, 2009).

Question: How long will it take glucose levels to decrease after the antipsychotic is stopped?

– Clinical experience shows that if the second-generation antipsychotic was associated with type II diabetes, it is likely to take a longer time to resolve.

– If the antipsychotic was associated with an acute onset of severe hyperglycemia/ diabetic ketoacidosis, it may be fatal, diabetes may persist after the diabetic ketoacidosis resolves (Polcwiartek et al., 2016; Cohen and Correll, 2009), or the hyperglycemia may resolve within one or two months in some cases.

Clinical recommendations

We should monitor patients for possible hyperglycemia EVEN IF they have not had significant weight gain since starting the antipsychotic. For recommendations on how to monitor patients for possible metabolic side effects in patients on a second-generation antipsychotic, please see the chapter on "Weight".

Resolution of hyperglycemia after switching to aripiprazole

In switching from atypicals, is there going to be a decrease in the severity of type II diabetes, e.g. fasting blood glucose? The patient was on risperidone and the blood sugar was running in the 150s to 180s. The patient was then switched to aripiprazole. How long would you give this before coming to the conclusion that the sugars aren't likely to come down?

As of May 2020, there are three published case series relevant to this question. Let's first look at what happened when these patients were switched from another antipsychotic to aripiprazole.

Case series 1

In one case series, nine patients were switched from another antipsychotic to aripiprazole after they developed diabetes (De Hert et al., 2006). The previous antipsychotics were quetiapine (two patients), risperidone (two patients), clozapine (one patient), olanzapine (one patient), and a first-generation antipsychotic (one patient).

All of them had impaired glucose tolerance in the oral glucose tolerance test and fasting glucose above 100 mg/dL. Three months after switching to aripiprazole, diabetes was reversed in all nine patients. Weight, waist circumference, and fasting insulin improved as well.

Case series 2

But, in another case series, patients of whom three-fourths were insulin resistant and about half had impaired or diabetic glucose tolerance while being treated with an antipsychotic were then switched to aripiprazole (Kim et al., 2007).

There was no improvement in weight, fasting glucose, lipids, and insulin resistance after being switched to aripiprazole.

Case series 3

In a third case series, seven patients with recent-onset diabetes and another six with prediabetes (impaired glucose tolerance or fasting glucose) were switched from their previous antipsychotic to aripiprazole (De Hert et al., 2007).

Three months after the switch to aripiprazole, all seven cases of diabetes had been reversed although one of the seven still had impaired glucose tolerance. Also, all six cases of prediabetes had resolved.

Bottom line

So, the answer to the question is (of course) that it "depends"— on how long the hyperglycemia had been present, how much weight the person had gained, whether the weight decreases after the switch to aripiprazole, etc, etc. But, I want to make two comments:

1. The hyperglycemia may or may not resolve after switching to aripiprazole. We cannot assume that switching the antipsychotic will be enough.

2. In cases where the hyperglycemia does improve after switching to aripiprazole, it may resolve within about three months.

Clinical recommendations

The following is my opinion, though based on the limited published data and on clinical experience:

– If we see the weight and fasting blood glucose slowly going down after switching to aripiprazole, we may continue to wait, hoping for further improvement.

– But, if after 3 or 4 months, we don't see any substantial improvement in weight and fasting glucose, I think it is unlikely that the diabetes will get reversed simply by the switch to aripiprazole.

– If treatment for type II diabetes it has not already been started earlier, it should be started now without further delay.

References: See https://simpleandpractical.com/side-effects-references

CHAPTER 12: LIVER

HYPERAMMONEMIA (ELEVATED AMMONIA LEVEL)

Valproate (Depakote®) and elevated serum ammonia level (hyperammonemia)

Valproate (divalproex; brand name Depakote) can be associated with an increase in serum ammonia (hyperammonemia). This can occur with carbamazepine as well.

[Optional to read: The mechanism of valproate-induced hyperammonemia is not clear. One of the mechanisms is that one of its metabolites interferes with the normal conversion of ammonia to urea, which would have been followed by excretion of the urea.]

Before jumping the gun

Before stopping the valproate or treating the hyperammonemia (as discussed below), it is important to first make sure it is not a false positive! (See this article: False-positive elevation of plasma ammonia). It is my impression that false-positive elevated serum ammonia results are quite common. This should not be surprising given the special handling of the blood sample needed to prevent a false-positive increase in serum ammonia. For details, please see this article: False-positive elevation of plasma ammonia).

Clinical features

Hyperammonemia can sometimes occur even in patients who have been on valproate for many years (e.g., Stewart, 2008).

The clinical presentation varies tremendously:

1. The patient may be asymptomatic.

2. It can present with symptoms like acute change in cognitive

functioning, lethargy, drowsiness, hypothermia, focal neurological symptoms, nausea/ vomiting, etc. When the patient is symptomatic, the condition is called valproate-induced hyperammonemic encephalopathy (VHE).

3. In severe cases, the hyperammonemia may be part of a syndrome of hepatic encephalopathy (confusion, hyperreflexia, asterixis or flapping tremor, vomiting, etc.).

Risk factors

Who is more likely to develop hyperammonemia on valproate? Here are a few of the risk factors. The first three of them are more likely to be encountered by mental health clinicians.

— Excessive alcohol use

— Combined use of valproate and topiramate

— Poor nutrition

— Urea cycle disorders, a group of rare, genetic disorders of urea metabolism

— Carnitine deficiency

— High protein intake

Do we need to routinely check serum ammonia?

The official Prescribing Information for divalproex (brand name Depakote ER) states: "…measure ammonia level if unexplained lethargy and vomiting or changes in mental status, and also with concomitant topiramate use…"

If a patient on divalproex is asymptomatic, we should ask ourselves whether we need to check the serum ammonia level. In my clinical practice, I use divalproex a lot and I never check serum ammonia unless the patient has mental confusion, lethargy, etc.

Evaluation

I want to repeat here for emphasis that the first step should be to verify that it was not a false-positive increase in serum ammonia due to the blood sample not being handled properly.

The most important thing, of course, is to check the hepatic function tests. Hyperammonemia may occur in isolation but it may also be one manifestation of potentially very serious liver damage.

Note: Serum valproic acid levels are not correlated with serum ammonia levels (Thomas et al., 2016) and are usually within the normal range in patients with valproate-associated hyperammonemia (Lewis et al., 2012).

Note: Hepatic (liver) function tests not only CAN be normal but usually ARE normal in these patients (Lewis et al., 2012).

We should not assume that valproate is the cause or the only cause of the elevated ammonia level. So, we should look for the following other possible causes of hyperammonemia. Here are just a few of them:

– Gastrointestinal bleeding. This is important to consider!

– Medications: diuretics, opioids, etc.

– Smoking

Management

If liver enzymes (AST, ALT) and/or bilirubin are significantly increased in a patient on valproate and the patient shows signs of encephalopathy, this should be considered a medical emergency and its management is not discussed here.

Instead, below, I will discuss how to approach patients on valproate whose hepatic function tests are normal (or only mildly abnormal) but the serum ammonia level is increased (hyperammonemia). I have divided the management into three categories based on the severity of the problem.

Note: If the patient is on both valproate and topiramate, stopping one of the two medications resolves the problem in most cases (Prescribing Information).

Level 1: Asymptomatic hyperammonemia

1. Several authors have continued the medication at the same dose or a lower dose even if serum ammonia is elevated. If the patient is asymptomatic and the increase in serum ammonia is relatively mild, we may consider continuing the valproate and simply monitoring the patient clinically and by periodically rechecking the serum ammonia level.

The Prescribing Information for divalproex (brand name Depakote ER) also does not recommend immediately stopping the valproate in cases where the serum ammonia is increased but the patient is asymptomatic. But, it recommends that "If the elevation persists, discontinuation of valproate therapy should be considered."

So, we don't necessarily have to stop the valproate or do anything other than monitoring the patient both clinically and by rechecking the serum ammonia level periodically.

2. What else can we do except monitoring the patient clinically and by repeatedly checking the serum ammonia levels?

Reducing the dose of the valproate has been found to significantly lower ammonia levels and may be considered.

3. Sometimes, due to more severe and persistent hyperammonemia, we may have to stop the valproate.

4. But, if continuing the valproate is thought to be very desirable, we can consider continuing the valproate and adding l-carnitine, lactulose, or both. This may lead to resolution of the asymptomatic hyperammonemia, allowing the valproate to be continued (e.g., Aiyer et al., 2016; Brown et al., 2018; Rousseau et al., 2009).

For a brief overview of l-carnitine, see this article: L-carnitine (levocarnitine): Basic information

Level 2: Mild valproate-induced hyperammonemic encephalopathy (VHE)

If the patient has significant symptoms of mental confusion, lethargy, etc., we should consider one or more of the following interventions.

1. Stop the medication, at least temporarily. The Prescribing Information for divalproex (brand name Depakote ER) recommends

stopping valproate if the ammonia level is increased and the patient is symptomatic.

2. Consider giving oral L-carnitine (levocarnitine; Brown et al., 2018; Mock and Schwetschenau, 2012; Lheureux and Hantson, 2009; Lheureux et al., 2005; Raskind et al., 2000)

3. If the VHE resolves after stopping the valproate and the valproate needs to be restarted, l-carnitine may be given along with it (e.g., Brown et al., 2018).

For a brief overview of l-carnitine, see this article: L-carnitine (levocarnitine): Basic information

Level 3: Severe valproate-induced hyperammonemic encephalopathy (VHE)

More severe cases of encephalopathy due to valproate-induced hyperammonemia will not be treated by the mental health clinician but we should know the main points.

– Lactulose is typically given in such cases.

– In severe cases, both L-carnitine and lactulose may be given.

– Other treatments that are sometimes considered include neomycin (Chopra et al., 2012).

Level 4: Hepatic encephalopathy

Here, along with the increased serum ammonia level, hepatic function tests are also significantly impaired. This is a medical emergency and mental health clinicians would not treat this condition. Its management is not discussed in this section.

False positive elevation of plasma ammonia

Valproate has been reported to be associated with asymptomatic elevations of plasma ammonia in some cases. So when plasma ammonia is elevated, patients may get taken off their divalproex. But wait! Are you sure if was not a false positive?

Ammonia levels increase spontaneously in blood and plasma after the sample has been collected. Why? Because ammonia is released from RBCs and because amino acids in the plasma get deaminated.

A consensus statement from a specialty group (Urea Cycle Disorders Conference group, 2001) suggested special measures for collecting blood for measurement of ammonia. These measures are also recommended by major US laboratories, e.g., Labcorp.

Sample collection instructions

Collection of the blood sample for measurement of plasma ammonia is tricky. Before we react to a report of elevated plasma ammonia in a patient who is asymptomatic, we should try to found out if the sample was properly collected and processed as per the guidelines below. Just glance over these instructions to get an idea of how much care needs to be taken!

1. The blood needs to be collected from a vein but without the use of a tourniquet because stasis of blood affects ammonia levels.

2. The patient should be instructed not to clench the fist, which is often done to make the veins prominent and to make blood collection easier. Muscular exertion can increase ammonia levels.

3. The patient should not have smoked prior to the blood draw because–guess what–smoking can increase ammonia levels.

4. The sample should be collected in a prechilled, ammonia-free tube.

5. The tubes in which the blood is collected should be filled completely and continuously kept tightly closed.

6. Now, here's the most special thing–As soon as the blood is drawn, it must be placed on ice.

7. The sample must be taken to the laboratory immediately.

8. Within 15 to 20 minutes after the blood is drawn, it must be centrifuged and the plasma separated.

9. If the test is not being done immediately, the plasma should immediately be frozen at $-70°C$.

Yeah, we better make sure before we overreact to mild increases in plasma ammonia.

References: See https://simpleandpractical.com/side-effects-references

CHAPTER 13: MOUTH

BRUXISM

What is bruxism?

Bruxism is involuntary clenching and/or grinding of the teeth. Contrary to popular belief, it can occur during the day ("wakeful bruxism", "awake bruxism", or "diurnal bruxism"), while asleep ("sleep bruxism" is a better term than "nocturnal bruxism"), or both.

Sleep bruxism is a form of parasomnia that occurs during non-REM sleep during which muscle tone is intact and movement can occur.

The mechanisms and treatment of awake bruxism and sleep bruxism may not be the same and so, pending further research, we should not assume that a treatment that works for sleep bruxism will invariably work for awake bruxism as well. Various medications affect either sleep bruxism, awake bruxism, or both (Falisi et al., 2014).

What are the consequences of bruxism?

It is important to not miss bruxism because it can cause serious damage to the teeth and also have a number of other negative effects.

Bruxism should be suspected if any of the following are present:

– Damage to the enamel of the teeth

– Pain in the teeth

– Fracture (crack, chip) of teeth

– Sensitive teeth

– Failure of dental restorations (fillings, crowns)

– Headache, e.g., bitemporal headache

– Pain and stiffness in the jaw muscles

– Pain and inflammation in the temporomandibular joint

– It can even lead to displacement of the temporomandibular joint (Falisi et al., 2014)!

– Impaired sleep in the person with bruxism and in the person sleeping in the same room

– Involuntary biting of the lip or cheek may also occur

What are the causes of bruxism?

1. Idiopathic

2. Anxiety, stress, anger, etc.

3. Sleep apnea

4. Parkinsonism and other movement disorders

5. Smoking may make it worse

4. Medications

Among psychotropic medications, it is most frequently associated with serotonergic antidepressants. One study suggested that the incidence of "antidepressant-induced bruxism" may be as high as 14% of patients taking an antidepressant (Uca et al., 2015).

In addition to antidepressants, bruxism may occur with methylphenidate, atomoxetine, antipsychotics, methadone, etc.

5. Substance abuse: Cocaine, methamphetamine, MDMA

Note: this is not a complete list of all possible causes of bruxism.

Management of antidepressant-induced bruxism

Before we get to discuss which medication can be added as an antidote for antidepressant-induced bruxism, let us discuss what else we can try first.

General measures

1. *Wait and watch?*

In some cases (e.g., Iskander et al., 2012), antidepressant-induced bruxism may subside on its own without any treatment. Similarly, it was reported to subside when the depression was treated with the addition of ECT to the antidepressant (Miyaoka et al., 2003).

However, it is not known how likely this kind of "spontaneous" improvement is or how long one should wait. I do not recommend waiting in severe cases or those with evidence of dental damage.

2. *Reducing the dose of the antidepressant, if possible, should be tried since this adverse effect (like most adverse effects) is dose-related.*

A case was reported of bruxism on escitalopram 40 mg/day (higher than the standard dose) that resolved completely when the dose was reduced to 25 mg/day (Ranjan et al., 2006).

Similarly, the same authors reported resolution of bruxism in another patient when venlafaxine was reduced from 225 mg/day to 187.5 mg/day (Ranjan et al., 2006).

3. *Take measures to reduce anxiety.*

Anxiety makes bruxism worse, so if significant anxiety is present, pharmacological or non-pharmacological measures (other than the antidepressant) should be employed to reduce the anxiety as much as possible.

4. *Switching to a different medication may or may not work.*

Switching the antidepressant, even within the same class, may sometimes resolve the bruxism (e.g., Chang et al., 2011). However, in other cases, bruxism occurs with a different antidepressant as well (e.g., Jaffee and Bostwick, 2000; Kuloglu et al., 2010).

So, the decision on whether to switch the medication or not may depend on factors other than the bruxism. For example, if the antidepressant has not worked very well but has led to bruxism, it makes sense to try a switch in the antidepressant for both reasons.

5. *If the problem persists, to prevent damage to the teeth, a night guard should be worn in the mouth while sleeping.*

Such night guards are available over-the-counter and this should suffice if we hope that the bruxism will soon resolve one way or the other. If for any reason, the bruxism lasts for longer, a custom nightguard may need to be made by a dentist.

6. *Since smoking makes bruxism worse, the person should be helped to reduce or stop smoking.*

7. *Ask the patient to see his or her dentist for evaluation and monitoring of the degree of damage to the teeth.*

Potential antidotes

No clinical trial of a pharmacological treatment of antidepressant-induced bruxism has been published as of March 2017. Zero. However, the following treatments have been found to work in case reports and clinical experience. Until formal studies are done, this is what we have to go on.

In published case reports, the antidote most frequently used in the treatment of antidepressant-induced bruxism is buspirone (Ellison and Stanziani, 1993: Romanelli et al., 1996; Bostwick and Jaffe, 1999; Jaffe and Bostwick, 2000; Wise, 2001; Pavlovic, 2004; Sabuncuoglu et al., 2009; Kuloglu et al., 2010; Çolak Sivri et al., 2016). Buspirone was also used successfully in a child to treat bruxism that was not due to a psychotropic medication (Orsagh-Yentis et al., 2011).

Therefore, I use this as the first-line treatment.

Other reasons why adding buspirone may be a good idea:

– Buspirone can augment the benefits of the antidepressant–for depression and for anxiety, and

– Buspirone can potentially treat antidepressant-induced sexual dysfunction if present (Landen et al., 1999).

Warning! When buspirone is added to a serotonergic medication, there is a risk of serotonin syndrome.

Buspirone: What dose? How long does it take to work?

Ellison and Stanziani (1993): I don't have this article yet.

Romanelli et al. (1996): I don't have this article yet.

Bostwick and Jaffee (1999): Buspirone 10 mg twice daily led, within one month, to full resolution of awake bruxism and bitemporal headaches that developed on sertraline 100 mg/day in a 35-year-old man.

Bostwick and Jaffee (1999): Buspirone 10 mg twice daily led within one week to improvement of sleep bruxism that had developed on sertraline 100 mg/day in a 64-year-old woman. Whether the dose was increased later and whether or not full resolution occurred later is not described in the paper.

Bostwick and Jaffee (1999): Buspirone 10 mg three times a day led to complete resolution within three weeks of bruxism (both awake and sleep) that had developed in a 38-year-old woman on sertraline 150 mg/day.

Bostwick and Jaffee (1999): Buspirone had to be titrated up to 50 mg/day to gradually achieve full relief of jaw tightness and constriction headache that occurred in a 32-year-old woman soon after starting sertraline and worsened as the sertraline was increased to 100 mg/day. This patient was able to taper off the buspirone after two months without the jaw tightness or headache recurring.

Jaffee and Bostwick (2000): Buspirone 10 mg twice daily improved bruxism in a 29-year-old woman on venlafaxine 150 mg/day, but further improvement occurred with each dose increase up to 30 mg twice daily. However, the bruxism did not resolve completely.

Jaffee and Bostwick (2000): In another case reported in the same paper, buspirone 10 mg twice daily was used in a 36-year-old woman on venlafaxine 75 mg/day. Full resolution occurred within 3 days of starting the buspirone.

Pavlovic (2004): Buspirone 40 mg/day was used to treat awake bruxism in a 64-year-old woman on venlafaxine 150 mg/day. After 4 weeks of treatment, it was noted that almost complete improvement occurred. However, the author did not describe whether the improvement had already occurred earlier than that.

Wise (2001): Addition of buspirone led to the cessation of bruxism that developed on citalopram 40 mg/day but no details were provided.

Sabuncuoglu et al. (2009): Buspirone 10 mg at bedtime was used in a 15-year-old girl on fluoxetine 20 mg/day. Full resolution occurred in about a week.

Kuloglu et al. (2010): Buspirone 20 mg/day was used in a 31-year-old woman on venlafaxine 150 mg/day. Full resolution occurred in about ten days.

Çolak Sivri et al. (2016): Buspirone 5 mg three times a day was used in a 7-year-old boy on fluoxetine 15 mg/day. Significant improvement occurred within 5 days and the bruxism was gone in about a week.

What do we conclude from these case reports?

I have reviewed the published case reports of using buspirone to treat antidepressant-induced bruxism and here are three simple principles that I found:

1. Buspirone may be given only at bedtime if it is only sleep bruxism. Otherwise, it can be given in either two or three doses per day.

2. The dose needed in adults is not very low. In adults, about 20 to 40 mg/day is likely to work. The dose used may be lower in children and adolescents.

3. A long trial is not needed. Improvement occurs within one or two weeks of starting buspirone (or of getting to the effective dose).

Note for academics only: the following case reports are not convincing and should not be considered:

Albayrak and Ekinci (2011): the buspirone was started after the duloxetine was stopped.

Milanlioglu (2012): the buspirone was started after the paroxetine was stopped.

Chatterjee et al. (2013): the buspirone was started after the paroxetine was stopped.

Mukherjee et al. (2014): a dose reduction was done with some benefit and then buspirone was added. It is not clear that the benefit was due to the buspirone rather than to the dose reduction.

Other medications have occasionally been reported to work for antidepressant-induced bruxism, but cannot be recommended at this time due to lack of sufficient experience with them. These include: gabapentin (Brown and Hong, 1999), low-dose aripiprazole (Oulis et al., 2012), and valproate (Lin and Tang, 2013)

Other treatments have been used for bruxism that is not caused by a psychotropic medication (e.g., amitriptyline, clonazepam, clonidine, botulinum toxin). These are not discussed here because we should not assume that all cases of bruxism are similar.

DRY MOUTH (XEROSTOMIA)

Medication-induced dry mouth (xerostomia)

Why is dry mouth important?

Dry mouth (or xerostomia if you want to speak in Latin to sound more impressive) is neglected most of the time, but it may not be a minor symptom. It can be quite important not only because it is uncomfortable but also because saliva protects the teeth, tongue, and mouth because saliva has antibacterial, buffering, and remineralization effects. So if a patient has dry mouth, he/she can develop dental caries or infection of the tongue/mouth. This problem can be compounded by the fact that patients with a depressive disorder may have worse self-care (including dental) behaviors than other persons.

In addition, dry mouth can lead to impairment in taste, inflammation of the mouth, inflammation of the gums, halitosis, dry lips, impaired fitting of dentures, impaired sleep, etc.

Which medications cause dry mouth?

Dry mouth can be caused by hundreds of medications. Psychotropic medications (from several different groups) are perhaps the most common culprits. Anticholinergic effects are not the only mechanisms by which psychotropic medications can cause dry mouth. The salivary glands are innervated by both the sympathetic and the parasympathetic nervous systems. For example, up to a third of patients on SSRIs have dry mouth.

Identifying dry mouth

The most important point is to ask all patients specifically about whether they have dry mouth.

I have become sensitized to observing patients for dry mouth and often pick it up when I notice that the patient is repeatedly licking his/her lips or squeezing the cheeks together.

Ask the patient to open the mouth while keeping the tongue in. Look for a normal small pool of saliva at the front of the mouth (under the tongue).

Ask the patient to protrude the tongue and see if it looks moist

Dry mouth (xerostomia): Management

Level 1 strategies

Avoid things that will dry the mouth further

— Alcohol-based mouthwash like Listerine

— Tobacco in any form

— Caffeine (as much as possible)

Oral Hygiene

If a patient has dry mouth, he/she needs to take MORE care of the teeth than other people.

– Brush the teeth at least twice a day, preferably three times a day

– Rinse the mouth out after every meal and every sugar-containing drink

– Floss every single day, even if he/she was not that regular in the past

– More frequent dental cleanings — every three months rather than every four months as is standard in the US. However, dental insurance pays for only two cleanings per year, so the patient has to be willing to pay out of pocket for the additional cleanings. Getting extra cleanings is wise when there is any increased risk for dental caries. For example, when children have braces, cleanings every three months are recommended as well.

Increasing saliva production

– Eating foods that stimulate production of saliva, like carrots, apples, and celery

– Using sugarless chewing gum or candy can stimulate saliva production. (Gum or candy with sugar in it must be avoided.)

Other measures

– Sipping small amounts of water frequently helps to some extent. However, the patient doesn't need to drink extra water. The body misinterprets dry mouth as thirst. If the urine is not yellow, the patient is drinking enough water.

– Sipping water or another beverage while eating can be helpful in swallowing food and may improve the taste of food.

– Sucking on ice chips can help with dry mouth

– Using a cool mist humidifier, day and night, and especially in the winter, should be considered because increasing moisture in the air can reduce dry mouth

Over-the-counter products

– The patient may need to use a group of special products called

Biotene (gel, oral rinse, gum, toothpaste, etc) that are available at all grocery stores and pharmacies and are not expensive. For example,

Biotene Oral Rinse

Biotene Oral Balance Dry Mouth Relief Moisturizing Gel, Long Lasting Saliva Substitute

– Other saliva substitutes/oral moisturizers like cellulose gum, glycerin (e.g., Oasis moisturizing mouth spray), Salivart®, Oralube®, Xero-lube®, etc.

– Xylitol-containing chewing gum may be particularly helpful. Xylitol is a sweetener used in some diabetic products that has special dental benefits. It is believe to reduce dental caries and may also help to remineralize enamel. Xylitol is taken up by bacteria by cannot be used by them, thus decreasing bacterial proliferation. Chewing gum with xylitol is available in a variety of brands including Spry, Epic, and Pur that are available in local pharmacies and on amazon.com. The gum must be used about six times a day for it to have full benefit. Six pieces of xylitol-containing gum would cost about 66 cents. Xylitol is also available in other forms like Orahealth XyliMelts that contain timed release xylitol, Xlear Spry Rain Oral Mist with Xylitol.

Xclear Spry Gum

Orahealth Xylimelts

Level 2 strategies

One measure that I have used at times is topical pilocarpine which minimizes systemic side effects.

Dry mouth (xerostomia) management: pilocarpine "mouthwash"

I'll discuss the off-label use of pilocarpine applied LOCALLY in the mouth.

The salivary glands secrete saliva in response to parasympathetic (cholinergic) stimulation. This is why medications with anticholinergic activity so frequently cause dry mouth.

The salivary glands secrete saliva in response to parasympathetic (cholinergic) stimulation. This is why medications with anticholinergic activity so frequently cause dry mouth. Pilocarpine is a cholinergic medication that can relieve dry mouth.

Oral pilocarpine can cause either tachycardia or bradycardia. It can also cause hypertension in 3% of patients compared to 1% of those on placebo.

But, to treat dry mouth, we only need a cholinergic effect in the mouth and not throughout the body, right?

Does it work?

Several, though not all, randomized, controlled clinical trials *that* compared topical pilocarpine to a placebo found it to be efficacious for increasing salivary flow and for decreasing subjective and objective evidence of dry mouth (Bernardi et al., 2002; Davies and Singer, 1994; Frydrych et al., 2002; Tanigawa et al., 2015; Cifuentes et al., 2018; Watanabe et al., 2018)

Note: These clinical trials were not conducted in psychotropic medication-induced dry mouth. They included patients with other causes of dry mouth, including Sjögren syndrome and radiation-induced dry mouth.

How to make a pilocarpine mouth wash

As of July 2020, pilocarpine is only available as a tablet or as eye drops, not as a topical spray. Some clinical trials used special formulations of pilocarpine to be used topically in the mouth. But, multiple clinical trials of pilocarpine "mouthwash" to treat dry mouth prepared the mouthwash by using pilocarpine eye drops (e.g., Frydrych et al., 2002; Kim et al., 2014) or pilocarpine tablets dissolved in water (e.g., Tanigawa et al., 2015).

Note: The concentration of topical pilocarpine varies greatly between studies from 0.01% (Tanigawa et al., 2015) to 1.5% (Pereira et al., 2020).

Note: Even though we call it a "mouthwash", a relatively small volume of the solution is enough to coat the inside of the mouth.

Using pilocarpine eye drops

The cost of generic pilocarpine eye drops has gone up significantly in the last few years. Cost-wise, it makes sense to use the 4% solution and dilute it.

Using pilocarpine tablets

Pilocarpine mouthwash can also be prepared by dissolving a 5 mg tablet of pilocarpine in tap water (e.g., Tanigawa et al., 2015). A patient may use three of the 5 mg tablets per day in this way. Of course, this does not at all mean that the patient will absorb anywhere near the amount of pilocarpine contained in the tablet; most of it will end up being spit out.

How to use the pilocarpine mouthwash

The pilocarpine solution can be used three or more times a day.

Patients may prefer to time the use of topical pilocarpine to when they feel they need it the most, e.g., before meals or before a social engagement in which the dry mouth would make it difficult to speak easily.

To get the greatest benefit from topical pilocarpine while also minimizing the potential side effects, the patient should be told that there are two key things that must be done:

1. Hold the pilocarpine in the mouth for one or, ideally, two minutes

2. After that, spit the solution out completely by spitting a few times. It is very important that the solution should not be swallowed because that would defeat the purpose of using the pilocarpine topically in the mouth.

Contraindications

It is very important to know that oral pilocarpine is contraindicated in patients with acute asthma, narrow-angle glaucoma, or iritis (Wiseman and Faulds, 1995).

Since at least some pilocarpine is absorbed into the body even from topical application in the mouth, and because a patient may swallow some or all of the pilocarpine mouthwash by mistake, patients with these conditions should also not be given topical pilocarpine.

Bottom line

Dry mouth can sometimes be quite bothersome and it greatly increases the risk of dental caries. Sometimes, it is essential to continue the medication that is causing the dry mouth but simpler options to manage the dry mouth do not work. In this difficult situation, expert psychopharmacologists can keep the off-label use of topical pilocarpine (pilocarpine "mouthwash") as a creative option for managing dry mouth.

Level 3 strategies: When all else fails

We do see patients in whom the dry mouth is not just a nuisance but also a torture and also a medical hazard, causing oral ulcers, caries, etc. Yet in some of these patients, the medication that is causing the dry mouth is thought to be life-saving. In such, thankfully rare, cases, when the simpler measures discussed above fail to provide relief, the use of an antidote should be considered.

It is useful for mental health clinicians to know that cevimeline (Evoxac®) and pilocarpine (Salagen®) are cholinergic medications that stimulate the salivary glands to increase salivary flow. While they have been studied in and are FDA approved for medical conditions with serious dry mouth (e.g., Sjögren's syndrome), their effects are non-specific and off-label use could be considered. However, they should only be prescribed by clinicians familiar with them. Others should consider referring their patient for a consultation.

HYPERSALIVATION (SIALORRHEA)

Clozapine-induced hypersalivation (sialorrhea)

Excessive salivation or sialorrhea is not only one of the commonest side effects of clozapine, it is very frustrating for patients, and we need to do more to identify it and to manage it.

But first, how common is it?

It occurs in about one-third of patients (sometimes reported in up to to 91% of patients) on clozapine and is one of the commonest adverse effects of clozapine (Bird et al., 2011).

Patients often don't report the hypersalivation to us, so we should specifically ask about it.

And, why is it such a big deal?

Hypersalivation can be quite bothersome to patients. It can result in:

– Waking up with a wet pillow.

– Impaired sleep. About a third of patients with hypersalivation are woken up at night because of it (Maher et al., 2016).

– Embarrassment

– Skin infection or maceration

– Swelling of the salivary glands, parotitis

– In extreme cases, aspiration and aspiration pneumonia.

Clinical features

(Bird et al., 2011)

– Develops early in the course of treatment

– Typically it is worse at night when the person is sleeping. However, daytime hypersalivation is also common, even if less so than at night.

– In contrast to most adverse effects, it is not dose related.

– It is unlikely to go away on its own if we just wait and watch
How can clozapine cause hypersalivation?

It may appear puzzling as to why clozapine, a medication known to have strong anticholinergic properties, should lead to hypersalivation. While the mechanism is not exactly known, it is believed to be related to the facts that clozapine:

1. While an antagonist at M3 mucarinic receptors, is an agonist at M4 mucarinic receptors.

2. Blocks alpha 1 and alpha 2 adrenergic receptors, leaving beta adrenergic receptors in the salivary glands unopposed, which increases saliva production.

Why should we bother to know these two hypothesized mechanisms of clozapine-induced sialorrhea? Because pharmacological treatments of this adverse effect are directed at these two mechanisms, as is discussed in the next section.

Clozapine-induced hypersalivation (sialorrhea): Treatment

General Measures

While most patients will need a medication to treat the hypersalivation, general measures can have some limited benefit.

– Titrating the clozapine up slowly may reduce the chances of developing sialorrhea.

– Even though the hypersalivation is not clearly dose related, reduction in the dose may be helpful in some cases, though it is probably not feasible for most patients given the importance of clozapine.

– If the patient is not already doing this, ask him or her to put a towel on this pillow to prevent the pillow from becoming drenched with saliva.

– For daytime hypersalivation, using sugarless chewing gum or candy encourages the person to swallow more often. Unfortunately, though, the hypersalivation is worst at night.

Oral anticholinergics–choose glycopyrrolate

While anticholinergic medications like benztropine and trihexyphenidyl are effective, I strongly recommend against using them for this purpose. Clozapine is a medication with significant anticholinergic properties. Adding another anticholinergic medication is likely to cause worsening of cognitive functioning.

Instead, I recommend using glycopyrrolate as the first line treatment. Glycopyrrolate is a nonselective blocker of muscarinic receptors. What are its advantages?

– It is a very potent blocker of M3 muscarinic receptors that are involved in salivation.

– It has a long duration of action in reducing salivary secretions, which is why it is often used prior to anesthesia.

– Most importantly, other anticholinergic medications cross the blood brain barrier and cause significant cognitive impairment. But glycopyrrolate does not cross into the brain to a significant extent. In a double-blind study comparing glycopyrrolate and biperiden (an anticholinergic), glycopyrrolate 1 mg twice daily did not worsen Mini Mental Status Examination scores while biperiden did (Liang et al., 2010).

– It is also less likely to cause cardiovascular adverse effects like arrhythmias.

– It is less likely to cause blurred vision.

– It is generic and cheap

Does it work?

Yes. It has been shown to be efficacious in a randomized, controlled trial (Liang et al., 2010).

What is the recommended dose?

The dose and the number of times the medication is given needs to be customized to the particular patient. Since usually the hypersalivation is worst at night, start with 1 mg given at bedtime. After 5 to 7 days, increase to 2 mg at night if needed. If there is hypersalivation during the day as well, another 1 mg can be taken in the morning and, if needed, in the afternoon.

Topical anticholinergics: choose ipratropium spray

What about giving anticholinergic medication locally in the mouth only? This could avoid the systemic side effects. Here are some options that have worked in case reports and chart reviews, though they have not been evaluated in systematic clinical trials:

While a drop of atropine 1% ophthalmic solution swished around in the mouth has been used, I recommend against using it because atropine is well absorbed across the mucous membranes of the mouth and can systemic and brain effects.

If a local treatment is used, we should consider using ipratropium 0.03% spray, one to two sprays sublingually. Ipratropium is a nonselective muscarinic blocker like atropine but is very poorly absorbed when given sublingually. If needed, it can be given three times a day. Also, if needed, a higher strength–0.06%–can be used.

The patient should be told clearly that even though the medication label will say that ipratropium is a nasal spray, we are recommending it for use in the mouth.

Note: the efficacy of ipratropium spray locally has not been established in systematic research. Case series and a large review of patient charts were strongly positive. Surprisingly, a small randomized, placebo-controlled trial (Sockalingam et al., 2009) did not show ipratropium spray 0.03% applied locally to be more efficacious than placebo. This may be because, in this study, there was a strong placebo response (40% of patients), making it hard to identify any potential benefit from ipratropium. Also, the higher strength was not tried. In my opinion, if a topical anticholinergic is to be tried, ipratropium spray is worth trying and has virtually no downside.

Other measures

While clonidine (case series by Praharaj et al., 2005) has been occasionally been used for the treatment of clozapine-induced hypersalivation, I don't recommend it because of the significant risk of additive hypotension.

References: See https://simpleandpractical.com/side-effects-references

CHAPTER 14: NERVOUS SYSTEM

AKATHISIA

Introduction

What is akathisia?

Akathisia is a very common, very bothersome, and potentially serious adverse effect of medications including antipsychotics, antidepressants, antiemetics, etc. It consists of a feeling of inner restlessness that is often but not necessarily accompanied by observable physical restlessness.

Why is akathisia so important?

1. It is common. Akathisia is not rare. With some medications, it is quite common. For example, in clinical trials of aripiprazole as an adjunctive treatment in patients with major depressive disorder, the drug-placebo difference for the incidence of akathisia was 21% (Abilify Prescribing Information). For brexpiprazole as an adjunctive treatment for MDD, the drug-placebo difference was 7% (Rexulti Prescribing Information). Note: the studies for aripiprazole and brexpiprazole were conducted differently, so these percentages should not be compared against each other.

2. Akathisia causes significant distress to the patient and so it can lead to non-adherence to the medication.

3. It can also lead to secondary effects like insomnia, aggressive behavior, and suicidality (Drake and Ehrlich, 1985).

4. It is believed that patients who have akathisia may be more likely to subsequently develop tardive dyskinesia.

Akathisia: Clinical features

Akathisia involves a subjective component assessed by asking the patient and an objective component assessed by observation.

The subjective component consists of inner restlessness that may be accompanied by anxiety, tension, impatience, irritability, etc. If a patient reports restlessness that is felt particularly in the legs, that is more suggestive of akathisia.

The objective component of akathisia consists of increased motor activity, for example, rocking from foot to foot, walking on the spot, rocking, fidgeting, pacing, and so on. The most characteristic motor symptoms of akathisia are rocking from foot to foot or walking on the spot when standing. These have been noted to occur in virtually all patients with moderate or severe akathisia. If a patient is rocking from foot to foot or walking on the spot and we still don't realize that the person has akathisia (which I have seen happen), that's not good! In severe cases of akathisia, patients may be unable to stand in one place without walking.

In mild cases, akathisia may be experienced only as inner restlessness, without any observable motor restlessness. In the majority of cases, however, the inner restlessness causes the patient to move around in an attempt to feel better. Conversely, objective signs suggestive of akathisia but without the subjective experience is called Pseudoakathisia.

Akathisia: Identification and evaluation

Assessing patients for possible akathisia

It is, unfortunately, not rare to misdiagnose akathisia as worsening of the underlying illness leading to the terrible error of increasing the dose of the antipsychotic rather than decreasing it. The key to identifying akathisia is to have a high index of suspicion for in all patients who present with motor restlessness, hyperactivity, or anxiety. Let me emphasize that: if you are not thinking of akathisia every time you see a patient who is restless, overactive, or anxious, you will definitely miss akathisia in some patients. On several occasions, I have seen patients who were identified by me as having akathisia that was missed by their previous psychiatrist. Very sad, because these patients unnecessarily suffered a lot and were in a bad shape when they came in to see me. They improved dramatically within a short period when the akathisia was identified and managed.

Examination for akathisia

The recommended assessment process is based on the Barnes Akathisia Rating Scale (BARS; Barnes, 1989, 2003). The BARS is useful for two reasons. One, it helps to guide the process of inquiry that helps to determine whether or not true akathisia is present. Two, using it, the clinician rates the severity of the akathisia which can both guide treatment at the time of examination and monitor change over time.

Step 1: Observation the patient when he/she does not know that he/she is being observed.

Step 2: For a minimum of two minutes, observe the patient specifically for akathisia while the patient is sitting

Step 3: For a minimum of two minutes, observe the patient specifically for akathisia while the patient is standing and talking to you about neutral topics.

Step 4: Ask patients if they have any of these:

- Inner restlessness and unease
- Whether the restlessness can be localized to any particular part of the body
- Awareness of difficulty sitting comfortably for long periods
- An urge to move
- Worsening on having to stay relatively still for long periods of time, especially while standing.
- Paresthesias (e.g., bugs crawling on the skin.)
- Pulling sensation in the muscles

If akathisia is present, ask about:

- Any diurnal variation of symptoms
- Awareness of any particular situations that seem to provoke or exacerbate the restlessness
- Any distress associated with the symptoms

Barnes Akathisia Rating Scale

The BARS is available for use at no cost by individual clinicians. The scale is reproduced below for study and the form (with appropriate copyright information included) may be downloaded at https://simpleandpractical.com.

Objective

0 Normal, occasional fidgety movements of the limbs

1 Presence of characteristic restless movements: shuffling or tramping movements of the legs/feet, or swinging of one leg, while sitting, and/or rocking from foot to foot

or 'walking on the spot' when standing, but movements present for less than half the time observed

2 Observed phenomena, as described in (1) above, which are present for at least half the observation period

3 The patient is constantly engaged in characteristic restless movements, and/or has the inability to remain seated or standing without walking or pacing, during the time observed.

Subjective

Awareness of restlessness

0 Absence of inner restlessness

1 Non-specific sense of inner restlessness

2 The patient is aware of an inability to keep the legs still, or a desire to move the legs, and/or complains of inner restlessness aggravated specifically by being required to stand still

3 Awareness of an intense compulsion to move most of the time and/or reports a strong desire to walk or pace most of the time

Distress related to restlessness

0 No distress

1 Mild

2 Moderate

3 Severe

Global clinical assessment of akathisia

0 Absent

No evidence of awareness of restlessness. Observation of characteristic movements of akathisia in the absence of a subjective report of inner restlessness or compulsive desire to move the legs should be classified as pseudoakathisia

1 Questionable

Non-specific inner tension and fidgety movements

2 Mild akathisia

Awareness of restlessness in the legs and/or inner restlessness worse when required to stand still. Fidgety movements resent, but characteristic restless movements of akathisia not necessarily observed. Condition causes little or no distress

3 Moderate akathisia

Awareness of restlessness as described for mild akathisia above, combined with characteristic restless movements

Akathisia: First-line treatments

The treatment chosen will depend on how severe the akathisia is and how important it is to continue on that particular medication. Here is a menu of options to choose from:

Prevent when possible!

Increase in the dose of the antipsychotic in the first few days of treatment is believed to be a risk factor for akathisia (Miller and

Fleischhacker, 2000). For example, rapid titration of risperidone was associated in one study with a more than six times greater odds of developing akathisia (Yoshimura et al., 2018. Note: in this study, for unclear reasons, rapid titration of aripiprazole did not increase the risk).

In my clinical experience, starting with a low dose and then gradually increasing the dose seems to very significantly reduce the incidence of akathisia.

Reduce the dose

Since akathisia is generally dose dependent, reduction of the dose should be considered, either alone or in conjunction with other strategies.

Wait-and-watch

Since akathisia is a very unpleasant symptom and can persist in many cases, waiting for the akathisia to resolve spontaneously is not recommended for most cases.

Changing the antipsychotic

Changing from one antipsychotic (e.g., aripiprazole) with a higher propensity to cause akathisia to another is a commonly used strategy that is often effective.

Treating the akathisia

In this section, let's discuss the most well-established and commonly used treatments for akathisia.

Propranolol

While the initial three very small trials (reviewed by Lima et al., 2004) did not provide clear evidence of propranolol's efficacy, a later randomized, controlled trial (Poyurovsky et al., 2006) in which propranolol was included as a control, did find it to be superior to placebo for treatment of akathisia. The dose of propranolol used in that study was 20 mg twice daily on day 1 and then 40 mg twice daily. But, long-acting propranolol (available as a generic, but the brand name is Inderal LA) can also be used and is available in 60 mg/day, 80 mg/day, 120 mg/day, and 160 mg/day strengths. The long-acting form is not expensive at all. But, what I typically do in my clinical practice is that I start with short-acting, plain propranolol, and once

I know that the person is tolerating it, I change to the long-acting form for convenience of use by the patient.

Contraindications to the use of propranolol include bronchial asthma, diabetes mellitus, cardiac conduction defects, and others. Its potential adverse effects include bradycardia, hypotension, and others. Please make sure to learn about propranolol before prescribing it.

On the other hand, metoprolol should not be considered as an alternative to propranolol for the treatment of akathisia because central effect and non-selective beta blockade seem to be required for an anti-akathisia effect (Miller and Fleischhacker, 2000). Metoprolol only becomes a non-selective beta blocker at high doses and at those high doses, it is associated with significant side effects. In short —we should not use metoprolol for akathisia. Also, we should not use beta blockers like atenolol that do not cross the blood-brain barrier readily and so are not centrally-acting.

Benzodiazepines

Two very small studies (reviewed by Lima et al., 2002) have supported the use of clonazepam in the treatment of akathisia.

Mirtazapine

Mirtazapine is, in my experience, a little-known treatment option for akathisia. Why mirtazapine? Because it is a potent 5-HT2A blocker and the pathophysiology of akathisia, though poorly understood, may be related in part to the ratio of 5-HT2A blockade to D2 blockade (Poyurovsky and Weizman, 2015). The use of mirtazapine is indirectly supported by the fact that other 5-HT2A antagonists may also work for akathisia, including trazodone (Stryjer et al., 2010), mianserin, and cyproheptadine.

A review of six clinical trials (Laoutidis and Luckhaus, 2014) concluded that 5-HT2A antagonists, including mirtazapine, are effective in the treatment of akathisia.

Two randomized, placebo-controlled studies (Poyurovsky et al., 2003, 2006; combined in the meta-analysis by Praharaj et al., 2015) found the addition of mirtazapine 15 mg/day to be efficacious for antipsychotic-induced akathisia. How effective was it? In one clinical trial, the percentage of responders (defined as a decrease of 2 or more points in the global score on the Barnes Akathisia Rating Scale at the last visit) were: mirtazapine

43%, propranolol 30%, placebo 7% (Poyurovsky et al., 2006). The drug-placebo difference between mirtazapine and placebo of 36% is huge!

The appeal of using mirtazapine instead of propranolol to treat akathisia is, of course, that it is easier and safer to use than propranolol because propranolol can be associated with hypotension and bradycardia. Also, the sedation from mirtazapine can help to reduce alleviating the anxiety and distress that comes with akathisia.

What about less than 15 mg per day? While the clinical trials of mirtazapine for the treatment of akathisia (Poyurovsky et al., 2003, 2006) used it in a 15 mg per day dose, it is possible that using 7.5 mg per day may be even better. We should keep in mind that mirtazapine is a potent blocker of 5-HT2A receptors at a low dose (Poyurovski and Weizman, 2015). A small retrospective case series reported mirtazapine 7.5 mg per day to be effective in treating akathisia with 41% patients responding to the treatment (Poyurovski and Weizman, 2018).

Does mirtazapine work better for akathisia due to a particular antipsychotic? This is not known, but if this is a possibility, I want to mention it here so that we clinicians can keep an eye out for this. In the one small retrospective case series of using mirtazapine 7.5 mg per day to treat antipsychotic-induced akathisia, mirtazapine was effective for 63% of patients in whom the akathisia was associated with aripiprazole but in only one of the four patients in whom the akathisia was associated with risperidone (Poyurovsky and Weizman, 2015). The authors noted that risperidone has a much higher ratio of 5-HT2A to D2 blockade than aripiprazole. So, they hypothesized that mirtazapine may be particularly useful for akathisia related to aripiprazole while akathisia related to risperidone use may need to be treated with propranolol. Again, I must emphasize that all this is unproven and speculative, but the clinical implication is so huge, that I thought it appropriate to mention it so that we clinicians can keep it at the back of our minds.

Mirtazapine may cause akathisia at higher doses

Important!

If we use mirtazapine for the treatment of akathisia, we should not increase the dose above 15 mg/day because, at higher doses, mirtazapine has also been reported to cause akathisia (Girishchandra et al., 2002;

Gulsun and Doruk, 2008). Note: very rarely, akathisia can also occur at 7.5 mg per day of mirtazapine (Koller, 2019).

How is this possible?

How could mirtazapine treat akathisia at low doses and cause akathisia at higher doses? This may be because at low doses, mirtazapine potently blocks 5-HT2A receptors but at higher doses blockade of alpha 2 receptors is more prominent (Poyurovsky et al., 2006). This hypothesis that alpha 2 blockade may make akathisia worse is supported by case reports that reported using clonidine, an alpha 2 agonist, to successfully treat akathisia (e.g., Zubenko et al., 1984; Amann et al., 1999).

How quickly does it start?

Well, in the reported cases, the akathisia occurred immediately (within hours) when the patient was started directly on mirtazapine 30 mg (Girishchandra et al., 2002; Gulsun and Doruk, 2008) or 15 mg (Raveendranathan and Swaminath, 2015), when the dose was increased from 15 mg to 30 mg (Girishchandra et al., 2002). But, it is not impossible for the akathisia to appear even after the patient has been on mirtazapine for years (Markoula et al., 2010).

Does it resolve?

The akathisia caused by mirtazapine resolved when:

1. The mirtazapine was stopped (Gulsun and Doruk, 2008)

2. The dose was reduced to 15 mg per day (Girishchandra et al., 2002).

3. Mirtazapine was continued at 30 mg but the akathisia was treated with clonazepam (Girishchandra et al., 2002)

4. Propranolol 20 mg was given daily along with the mirtazapine until the patient got used to the mirtazapine (Koller, 2019).

Gabapentin for the treatment of akathisia?

Medication-induced akathisia is a horrible side effect that can be difficult to treat. There are no FDA-approved treatments for akathisia, but centrally-acting beta blockers like propranolol, benzodiazepines, and low-dose mirtazapine are the best-established treatments. Is gabapentin another of the less studied, second-line treatment options?

Does it work?

Note: gabapentin is not only not FDA-approved for the treatment of akathisia (no medication is), it also has not been studied for the treatment of akathisia in a randomized, controlled clinical trial as of January 2019.

But, gabapentin has been used as an off-label treatment for akathisia in case reports and an open-label study. Its potential use for the treatment of akathisia is also supported indirectly by the appearance of akathisia during gabapentin withdrawal (See et al., 2011).

What dose of gabapentin?

This has varied greatly:

300 mg/day (open-label study by Takeshima et al., 2018b)

450 mg/day (case report by Takeshima et al., 2018a)

600 mg/day (case report by Takeshima et al., 2018a; open-label study by Takeshima et al., 2018b)

1200 mg/day (case report by Sullivan and Wilbur, 2014), and

3000 mg/day (case report by Pfeffer et al., 2005).

Anticholinergics for the treatment of akathisia?

It is very common to refer to akathisia to be lumped together with other movement disorders like medication-induced parkinsonism into a category of "extrapyramidal symptoms." This then leads to clinicians prescribing anticholinergic medications like benztropine (brand name Cogentin) for the treatment of akathisia. I have been seeing this for many years and have tried to address this question whenever I do talks about the management of side effects.

Do anticholinergic medications work for akathisia?

The use of anticholinergics for the treatment of akathisia is not supported by well-designed randomized controlled trials (Rathbone and Soares-Weiser, 2006). But, let's look at what data we do have from randomized, controlled clinical trials (RCTs).

1. A small RCT found benztropine 6 mg/day to be more effective than placebo for antipsychotic-induced akathisia but about a third of patients became confused or forgetful (Adler et al., 1993).

2. Intramuscular biperiden versus placebo repeated up to three times if needed (15 patients in each group)–no difference between biperiden and placebo (Baskak et al., 2007).

This should not be surprising because the mechanism by which akathisia occurs appears to be different from the mechanism responsible for other extrapyramidal symptoms.

Diphenhydramine (brand name Benadryl)?

In case anyone comes upon this study, a retrospective chart review found that diphenhydramine given along with prochloperazine for nausea reduced the incidence of akathisia (Vinson and Drotts, 2001). But, diphenhydramine was sedating for these patients. That's why, even though diphenhydramine has both antihistaminic and weak anticholinergic activity, this study cannot be taken as evidence that anticholinergics are effective for preventing medication-induced akathisia. Also, a large randomized controlled clinical trial of diphenhydramine for preventing metoclopramide-induced akathisia did not find any benefit of diphenhydramine.

Bottomline

Contrary to common clinical practice that I have noted, anticholinergic medications should not be used as first-line treatments for the treatment of akathisia.

Amantadine for the treatment of akathisia?

Amantadine 100 to 200 mg/day has been used off-label as a treatment for akathisia, but this has not been well studied.

Also, tolerance can develop rapidly (Zubenko et al., 1984).

So, I do not recommend its use for akathisia.

HEADACHE

Lamotrigine and headache

In data from short-term studies described in the Prescribing Information, headache did not occur twice as often as with placebo. So, we could not say with some confidence that the headache was likely to really be due to the lamotrigine.

On the other hand, many published studies reported headache to be a common side effect of lamotrigine in patients with epilepsy (Theis et al., 2005; Shechter et al., 2005; Sander et al., 1990). In fact, it was reported to be the commonest side effect of lamotrigine in patients with bipolar disorders (Bowden et al., 2004). And, headache is not necessarily a mild, nuisance side effect. In long-term treatment of epilepsy, headache is one of the common reasons given for stopping the medication (Faught et al., 2004)

This contradiction is an example of how screwed up the methodology of research on side effects is (Mago, 2016).

When statistical testing is done to compare the incidence of headache on lamotrigine versus on placebo, one study did not find the difference to be statistically significant (Giorgi et al., 2001). Similarly, a placebo-controlled study of high dose lamotrigine found that headache occurred equally on lamotrigine and on placebo (Matsuo et al., 1996).

Here are some more things to know about headache in a patient on lamotrigine.

– Headache occurs more commonly with combination therapy (e.g., with oxcarbazepine) than with monotherapy (Theis et al., 2005).

– Warning! If a patient on lamotrigine develops headache along with fever, nausea, and vomiting, we must suspect aseptic meningitis. These patients may or may not also have photophobia and a stiff neck.

PARKINSONISM

Can we prevent neuroleptic-induced parkinsonism?

Of course, the primary strategy to reduce the incidence of neuroleptic-induced parkinsonism is to choose an antipsychotic with a lower risk of parkinsonism.

But, what about for a given antipsychotic? Is there a way to reduce the incidence of parkinsonism (other than to give an anticholinergic medication prophylactically, which is usually not recommended; Barnes et al., 2011)?

Note the two facts listed below and see what conclusion they logically lead to:

1. The appearance of neuroleptic-induced parkinsonism suggests the dose may be too high.

2. In contrast to acute dystonias, neuroleptic-induced parkinsonism typically starts slowly—over several days or weeks (Hasan et al., 2013; Stroup and Gray, 2018).

When possible, we should titrate the antipsychotic up stepwise and slowly (Hasan et al., 2013). If, as the antipsychotic is being titrated up, parkinsonism begins to appear, this generally suggests that we should try to avoid increasing the dose further.

Does dose reduction work for neuroleptic-induced

parkinsonism?

The first step in managing neuroleptic-induced parkinsonism (the term used by DSM-5) should usually be to reduce the dose of the antipsychotic if possible (Hasan et al., 2013; Stroup and Gray, 2018) before considering the next steps:

Step 2: Switch, if possible, to an antipsychotic with a lower risk of parkinsonism

Step 3: Consider adding an anticholinergic medication (e.g., benztropine, trihexyphenidyl)

Step 4: Consider adding amantadine

Decrease by how much?

A small decrease in the dose may be all that is needed (Mamo et al., 1999); say, about 10%.

How long will it take to help?

Lowering the dose of the antipsychotic often helps reduce the parkinsonism relatively quickly—within a few days—but this may depend on the half-life of the medication.

Why might dose reduction help?

Except for clozapine and quetiapine, the antipsychotic efficacy of medications is generally correlated with increasing D2/D3 receptor occupancy (Yilmaz et al., 2012). But, only up to a point.

There seems to be a "therapeutic window" in terms of striatal dopamine D2/D3 receptor occupancy of approximately 60% to 80% as seen on PET scanning (Nord and Farde, 2011; Uchida et al., 2011, 2014).

What we mean by "therapeutic window" is that below about 60 to 65% occupancy of striatal D2/D3 receptors by the antipsychotic drug, the antipsychotic effect tends to not be optimal. On the other hand, when the antipsychotic drug occupies more than about 80% of the striatal D2/D3 receptors, extrapyramidal side effects are much more likely to occur (Kapur and Seeman, 2001).

This is presumably why dose reduction tends to reduce extrapyramidal side effects in many (though not all) patients (e.g., Uchida et al., 2014).

AMANTADINE FOR ANTIPSYCHOTIC-INDUCED PARKINSONISM

Question from a colleague: A patient of mine has EPS and isn't tolerating trihexyphenidyl well (says he's foggy headed, constipated and has dry mouth). He also has had problems with benztropine. I was thinking of trying amantadine but have never used it for EPS. Is this a medication you've found effective? If so, how do you dose it?

A note on terminology

I'll use the term "parkinsonism" to describe these side effects of antipsychotics rather than "extrapyramidal symptoms (EPS)" because akathisia is often included in the term EPS even though its pathophysiology and treatment are quite different.

What is amantadine?

Amantadine is a dopaminergic medication whose exact mechanism of action is not known. Its FDA indications are for:

1. Treatment of Parkinson's disease, parkinsonism due to other causes, and drug-induced extrapyramidal reactions.

2. Treatment of influenza type A.

In mental health, it has many other potential off-label uses.

Consider amantadine?

While anticholinergic medications are the first-line treatments for antipsychotic-induced parkinsonism when an antidote is needed, they can certainly have many side effects as in this patient. I agree that amantadine should be considered in this patient.

Amantadine is generally as effective as anticholinergics as a treatment for antipsychotic-induced parkinsonism.

If needed, it can be used along with an anticholinergic medication, though this combination can lead to increased anticholinergic side effects (see below).

Next, let's discuss some potential advantages and disadvantages of amantadine so that we can better understand its proper place in the treatment of antipsychotic-induced parkinsonism.

Advantages of amantadine

– Unlike anticholinergic medications, it does not cause memory impairment (McEvoy, 1987; Gelenberg et al., 1989).

– It is excreted unchanged and so is unlikely to be involved in any pharmacokinetic drug-drug interactions. But, see below for some possible drug interactions.

– It is generic and inexpensive.

It may also treat other antipsychotic adverse effects that may be present:

– It may also be effective for antipsychotic-induced weight gain (Graham et al., 2005; Zheng et al., 2017).

– It may also reduce prolactin levels if hyperprolactinemia is also present (Siever, 1981).

-It may also be effective for tardive dyskinesia for which it is a second-line option in the short term (Bhidayasiri et al., 2006; Angus et al., 1997; Pappa et al., 2010).

Disadvantages of amantadine

– Tolerance may develop over time, even after just a few weeks. This is more likely to happen with amantadine than with anticholinergics.

– It can precipitate mania, especially in patients with bipolar disorder (e.g., Rego and Giller, 1989; Sodré et al., 2010).

– It can worsen psychotic symptoms though this does not usually occur if the patient is on an adequate dose of an antipsychotic.

Dose (for antipsychotic-induced parkinsonism)

Usually, we start with 100 mg twice daily. If the symptoms are mild, we may even start with 100 mg once a day.

After at least 5 to 7 days, if symptoms are not adequately controlled, we can consider increasing the dose to 100 mg three times a day.

SEIZURES

Antidepressants and seizures

In one study (Wu et al., 2017), the odds ratios for the risk of a new-onset seizure with different antidepressant were:

Bupropion 2.23

Selective serotonin reuptake inhibitors (SSRIs) 1.76

Serotonin and norepinephrine reuptake inhibitors (SNRIs) 1.40

Mirtazapine 1.38

In this study, the increased risk of a new-onset seizure was greatest in the age group of 10 to 24 years.

Bupropion and seizures (part one): What clinicians need to know

In my experience, prescribing clinicians fall under two groups—those who are overly concerned about the seizure risk with bupropion and those who are hardly concerned—and I think both viewpoints are not consistent with the facts.

Bupropion is a valuable antidepressant because it does not cause sexual dysfunction or weight gain any more than placebo, can actually improve sexual desire, and can be energizing. We must correctly understand the seizure risk with bupropion so that we can prescribe it appropriately and can honestly tell patients what the degree of risk is.

Below, ladies and gentlemen, let us separate the facts and the myths about the role of dose and the preparation (immediate-release, sustained-release, or extended-release) in the association between bupropion and risk of seizures. In a separate article, I will discuss the role of other risk factors including comorbid illness, drug interactions, concomitant medications, and genetic polymorphisms.

1. The risk of a seizure with bupropion sustained-release preparation up to 300 mg/day is 0.1%, which is exactly the same as the risk with SSRIs. Thus, at this dose, it is not true (at doses up to 300 mg/day), as is commonly believed, that bupropion has a higher risk of seizures than the SSRIs.

2. The risk of a new-onset seizure in the general population is 0.08%, so the risk with SSRIs or bupropion sustained-release up to 300 mg/day is at the most only minimally greater than that in the general population (0.1% vs. 0.08%).

3. On the other hand, the risk of seizures with tricyclic antidepressants is 1% or ten times that with SSRIs or with bupropion sustained-release up to 300 mg/day.

4. What about the risk of seizures with bupropion sustained-release 400 mg/day? The risk is 0.4% (Prescribing Information) or four times greater than at doses up to 300 mg/day. So, the risk goes up once we use more than 300 mg/day. When using a dose greater than 300 mg/day is when we definitely need to tell patients about this elevated risk and to obtain informed consent.

Optional to read: It is unfortunate that the FDA and manufacturer have not worded their statements to be very clear either way about how the 0.4% number was arrived at. But, here's why I think it doesn't matter:

– The "official" document is the Prescribing Information and it states that bupropion sustained-release 400 mg/day is associated with a 0.4% risk of new-onset seizures. Whether arrived at directly or indirectly, that is the number that was decided on.

– With rare events and especially with a dose (400 mg/day) that is much less commonly used than 300 mg/day, it is impossible to have an exact number. Even one more person with a seizure would alter the percentage for the incidence.

– Since lower doses are much more commonly used, we are more confident that the risk with doses of bupropion sustained-release up to 300 mg/day is about 0.1%.

– The risk of seizures is definitely dose-related. (Also, by the way, some data suggest that the increase may not be linear. That is, it may rise more sharply after some threshold dose is reached.)Even though I do believe that the risk is less with sustained-release and extended-release preparations, this does not mean that with these preparations, serum levels don't go up as the dose increases.

– So, I find it impossible to believe that the risk of seizures is not MORE with 400 mg per day than it is with 150 to 300 mg/day. So, I would deduce that the risk of seizures with 400 mg/day is more than 0.1%. Whether it is 0.2% or 0.3% or 0.4%, we are not as sure.

– What is the practical point? Why are we even discussing this? It is that the risk of seizures is higher with higher doses and when other risk factors for seizures are present, we need to take this fact into account when deciding whether or not to go to a higher dose.]

5. I would urge you strongly to not prescribe bupropion doses greater than the recommended doses unless you have particular expertise in doing so and give an antiepileptic medication along with the bupropion. The risk of seizures increases ten-fold above 450 mg/day to 4%, which is unacceptably high.

6. Isn't the risk of seizures different depending on which preparation is used? There is little doubt that the immediate-release preparation has a higher risk of seizures compared to the sustained-release preparation. The incidence of seizures with bupropion went down dramatically when the sustained-release preparation was introduced (in 1996). While the immediate-release preparation is still available, we should avoid using it.

7. The risk of seizures is also dependent on the milligrams of bupropion given at one time. We must not prescribe more than 200 mg of bupropion sustained-release at a time (i.e., in one dose). On the other hand, bupropion extended-release can be given as 450 mg in a single dose, which is convenient.

8. What about sustained-release bupropion versus extended-release bupropion? There are no large comparative studies to answer that question definitely. There are at least two published cases of seizures on bupropion XL, but the clinical trials of XL had no seizures. So, I'm not completely sure whether the risk of seizures with bupropion extended-release is less than that with bupropion sustained-release. However, in general, I think that extended-release preparations have fewer adverse effects, so I always prescribe the extended-release preparation rather than the sustained-release preparation. Both are now available as generics in the US, so the cost difference is small.

9. What about risk of seizure in cases of overdose on bupropion? In persons who overdosed on bupropion XL (600 mg or more), 32% had a seizure. This further confirms to me that it not a myth that bupropion is associated with risk of seizures. This also tells us that we must be very cautious in prescribing bupropion to persons who may be at elevated risk of overdosing on the medication.

What factors can increase risk of seizures with bupropion?

We need to clearly know the risk factors that increase the risk of seizures with bupropion so that we can:

- Quickly and efficiently check for them in every person whom we start on bupropion, and

- Remain vigilant for on an ongoing basis.

(Interestingly, risk of seizures with bupropion is not a boxed warning ("black box warning") in the Prescribing Information. It is listed in the section on "Warnings," a lower level of concern.)

In the previous section we discussed:

1. The percentage of persons on bupropion who have new onset seizures.

2. The role of the dose of bupropion in modifying the risk: total dose per day, dose given at one time, rate of titration

3. The role of the particular preparation used in modifying the risk: immediate-release, sustained-release, extended-release

Next, I want to make some general points about dealing with these issues:

1. The official Prescribing Information and standard medical literature make recommendations about what to do and not to do. Of course, clinicians can choose to not follow one or more recommendations. However, in such cases, the prescribing clinicians must be prepared to defend themselves if they do not follow the recommendations and the patient has a seizure—whether or not the seizure was really due to the bupropion.

2. Even if a person does not have any of these risk factors, one of them can emerge later in treatment, even years later. For example, a new medication, a head injury, benzodiazepine dependence with risk of withdrawal, etc.

3. If a person has significantly increased risk for a seizure with bupropion but bupropion is thought to be essential or very helpful, off label use of a combination of bupropion and an antiepileptic is sometimes done. Advanced point: among these, phenytoin and carbamazepine also lower the levels of bupropion and may decrease its efficacy unless the dose of bupropion is increased.

Here are some other risk factors that may also increase risk of seizures with bupropion. We must systematically evaluate patients for these risk factors before starting bupropion and document that we did so.

Other mental disorders

According to the official Prescribing Information, bupropion is contraindicated in persons with a "current or prior diagnosis of bulimia or anorexia nervosa."

We should note that the contraindication includes:

– Both a current and a past diagnosis, and

– Both bulimia and anorexia.

It is often questioned whether this contraindication needs to be so black and white, but I am unaware of any research to back up the claim that bulimia and anorexia do not significantly increase the risk of seizures. So, at least for now, it stands as it is.

Other non-psychiatric medical disorders

1. Bupropion is contraindicated in patients with a history of seizure disorder. However, a history of febrile seizures in infancy should not be considered a contraindication.

2. History of severe head injury. It would not be reasonable to exclude everyone who had even a mild head injury. Besides asking how the head injury occurred and what treatment was required, one simple question to also ask is whether the person lost consciousness and, if so, for how long.

3. Other intracranial diseases like arteriovenous malformation, CNS tumor, CNS infection, severe stroke.

4. Metabolic disorders (e.g., hypoglycemia, hyponatremia, severe hepatic impairment, and hypoxia)

Substance use disorders: Risk of withdrawal

Bupropion is contraindicated in "abrupt discontinuation of alcohol, benzodiazepines, barbiturates, antiepileptic drugs." The main practical implication of this is that we should avoid bupropion in patients who are currently significantly physically dependent on alcohol, benzodiazepines, and other sedatives and may unexpectedly suffer from withdrawal symptoms and be at increased risk of seizures.

Substance use disorders: Additive risk

For a different reason than the one above, we should also avoid bupropion in persons who are currently actively abusing stimulants or cocaine because of additive seizure risk if such substances are combined with bupropion.

Concomitant medications: Increased levels

Bupropion is metabolized by cytochrome P450 isoenzyme 2B6. Note: 2 "B for boy" 6, not the 2D6 enzyme that we are much more familiar with.

CYP450 2B6 is inhibited by some medications that are commonly used: clopidogrel (Plavix®), ticlopidine (Ticlid®). Use of these medications along with bupropion may raise bupropion levels and increase risk of seizures. Other medications that inhibit CYP 450 2B6 are: thiotepa, voriconazole.

Concomitant medications: Additive seizure risk

1. Stimulants. We need to keep this increased risk in mind because stimulants and bupropion are often used together because bupropion is sometimes used off label as a treatment for ADHD or is used, rightly or wrongly, for concomitant "depression."

2. Tramadol

3. Clozapine

4. Tricyclic antidepressants

5. Diabetes mellitus treated with oral hypoglycemic drugs or insulin

6. Systemic steroids

7. Other medications that lower seizure risk

Genetic polymorphisms

Polymorphisms (variations) in the gene that codes for the cytochrome P450 isoenzyme 2B6 can now be easily tested for clinically, at least in the US. Poor metabolizer status for CYP 2B6 will increase the serum levels of bupropion.

Pharmacogenetic testing for predicted CYP450 2B6 metabolizer status is not a standard recommendation, but in my opinion a good idea when using more than 300 mg/day of bupropion or if other risk factors for seizures are present.

Testing for the CYP450 2B6 gene alleles is a standard part of two of the pharmacogenetic test batteries that are used in the US—the Genecept assay (Genomind, Inc) and the GeneSight assay (Assurex Health).

Clozapine and seizures

Clozapine has a unique position in psychiatry due to being the most efficacious antipsychotic. It sometimes works when no other antipsychotic has worked. However, among the second-generation antipsychotics, clozapine also has the highest risk of seizures. Here are some key things that prescribing clinicians need to know about clozapine and seizures.

1. Risk of seizures in persons on clozapine

According to the manufacturer, the cumulative risk of seizures over the first year of treatment can be as high as 5%. That's is really high, isn't it?

2. Risk continues to increase over the years

In contrast to many other adverse effects that tend to occur early in treatment, it is not true that the risk of seizures associated with clozapine is limited to the first few months.

Rather, the cumulative risk of seizures increases over the years.

3. Dose-dependent

The risk of seizures in persons on different doses of clozapine is as follows.

– Less than 300 mg/day—about 1%
– 300 to 599 mg/day—about 3%
– 600 mg/day or greater—about 4%

We can see from these numbers that:

– The risk of seizures with clozapine is dose-dependent though really it is the serum level that matters (see below).

– But even at a relatively low dose, the risk of seizures is much more than the baseline risk (which is about 0.1% or less).

4. Risk varies with serum level

More than the dose, the risk of seizures depends on the serum level of clozapine. A serum level greater than 600 ng/mL is associated with a higher risk of seizures.

However, unfortunately, seizures can occur at times even at therapeutic clozapine levels

5. *Increased risk with rapid titration*

Seizures are more common early in treatment with clozapine (Varma et al., 2011). So, while has not been clearly shown that slow titration of clozapine decreases the risk of seizures with clozapine, rapid titration is not advisable.

6. *What kind of seizures?*

While tonic-clonic seizures are the most common type of seizures that occur with clozapine.

But, myoclonic, atonic, or partial (simple or complex), and absence seizures should not be missed (Wong and Delva, 2007).

Myoclonic jerks usually present as orofacial movements, knee buckling, or leg folding (de Leon, 2014).

7. *What to tell patients*

The Prescribing Information states:

– "Inform patients and caregivers about the significant risk of seizure during CLOZARIL treatment."

– "Because of the substantial risk of seizure associated with CLOZARIL use, caution patients about engaging in any activity where sudden loss of consciousness could cause serious risk to themselves or others (e.g., driving an automobile, operating complex machinery, swimming, climbing)."

8. *Stop clozapine?*

In most cases, the occurrence of a seizure does not automatically mean that clozapine should be stopped (Nielsen et al., 2013). Measures can usually be taken to avoid further seizures.

9. *Which antiepileptic?*

In cases where clozapine is essential for a particular patient, even after a seizure has occurred, an antiepileptic medication is sometimes used along with clozapine to allow it to be continued and to be used in higher doses.

Which antiepileptic should we use?

Carbamazepine can decrease clozapine levels and also it is not recommended with clozapine because of possible additive effects in causing agranulocytosis.

Phenytoin can decrease clozapine levels significantly (two to four times) and careful management through serial measurement of clozapine levels would be needed if phenytoin was used.

Divalproex is probably the drug of choice for use with clozapine (Williams and Park, 2015). However, in rare cases divalproex may also increase or decrease clozapine levels and measurement of the clozapine level after addition of divalproex should be considered (de Leon, 2014).

Lamotrigine may occasionally be considered (e.g., Muzyk et al., 2010) but this may depend on the type of seizures. Lamotrigine is not indicated as monotherapy for generalized tonic-clonic seizures which are the commonest type of seizures associated with clozapine.

The mental health clinician must work in consultation with a neurologist to take this decision.

10. *Antiepileptic preventively, even before a seizure has occurred?*

Preventive treatment with an antiepileptic may be considered under certain circumstances (Varma et al., 2011):

– Serum clozapine level is more than 500 mcg/L

– Myoclonic jerks are present

– Other factors that increase the risk of seizures (e.g., a medication) are present, or

– The EEG shows clear epileptiform discharges. Note: EEG is not recommended or required. This refers to an EEG if done for any reason, so it will be rare that an EEG is available.

TARDIVE DYSKINESIA

Antidepressant-induced tardive dyskinesia

There have been occasional published reports of choreoathetoid movements (just like the tardive dyskinesia that occurs with dopamine receptor blockers) that occurred in persons who took an SSRI, SNRI, or tricyclic antidepressant but had never taken a dopamine blocking drug. There have also been over 200 unpublished reports of dyskinesias associated with the use of an antidepressant.

Other movement disorders (akathisia, dystonia, parkinsonism) have also been reported with antidepressants. This makes us more likely to believe that tardive dyskinesia can occur with antidepressants.

Tardive dyskinesia has also been reported in rare cases with lithium.

Risk factors

Tardive dyskinesia associated with antidepressant use is more likely to occur in older persons, such as the one described by our colleague.

Since dyskinesias can occur spontaneously, especially in older persons, it can sometimes be hard to be sure that the antidepressant was, in fact, the cause of the dyskinesia.

In many but not all of the patients who developed tardive dyskinesia on an antidepressant, there was a history of using an antipsychotic in the past.

Tardive dyskinesia: risk with second-generation (atypical) antipsychotics

Is the risk of TD with second-generation ("atypical") antipsychotics really lower than that with first-generation ("typical") antipsychotics?

Or was this a misleading claim by pharmaceutical companies that manufactured the much more expensive second-generation antipsychotics?

This question is of great clinical importance because we need to tell patients about the risk and to consider it in deciding which medication to give. The research on TD is confusing. But, here are some key points:

1. The risk of TD depends a lot on the age group being studied. So, we should look at each age group separately.

For example, a review of multiple studies of TD in older adults concluded that the incidence of TD was three times lower in older adults receiving a second-generation antipsychotic versus in those receiving a first-generation antipsychotic (23% versus 7% after one year of treatment; O'Brien, 2016).

2. Another study found that in patients who were at high risk of developing TD because they already had borderline dyskinesia, those treated with a first-generation antipsychotic were twice as likely to later develop definite TD as those treated with a second-generation antipsychotic (Dolder and Jeste, 2003).

3. Have those of you who practiced before there were second-generation antipsychotics noted any marked change in the number of patients with TD? Before second-generation antipsychotics, I used to see several patients with TD every day and this has markedly changed since the move to second-generation antipsychotics.

Potential mechanism

It is hypothesized that increased serotonergic activity inhibits dopaminergic neurotransmission in the striatum. That is, that serotonergic antidepressants indirectly have an antidopaminergic effect.

Management and prognosis

Tapered withdrawal of the antidepressant is probably wise. However, after stopping the antidepressant, the tardive dyskinesia may resolve, improve but not resolve, remain the same, or even worsen (Gerber and Lynd, 1998).

One review of the case reports noted that, as is true of antipsychotic-induced tardive dyskinesia, most cases of antidepressant-induced tardive dyskinesia did not improve after stopping the medication (Leo, 1996).

It has been theoretically speculated that sertraline may be less likely to cause tardive dyskinesia because, in addition to inhibiting serotonin reuptake, it also blocks dopamine reuptake to a greater extent than the other SSRIs (Leo, 1996). However, we don't have any data to support recommending that if an antidepressant medication is unavoidable, sertraline should be preferred.

While there is no reliable data on the treatment of antidepressant-induced tardive dyskinesia, for antidepressant-induced movement disorders, some of the same medications can be tried that are used for antipsychotic-induced movement disorders.

How EXACTLY to screen for tardive dyskinesia

Prescribers of antipsychotic medications know that it is essential to actively screen for tardive dyskinesia (TD) in all patients who are being treated with any antipsychotic medication. But, a question we receive frequently is: How often should we do the Abnormal Involuntary Movement Scale (AIMS)? So, let's go over exactly how to screen for TD, including how often to do an AIMS examination.

Our recommendations for how exactly to screen for tardive dyskinesia are based on:

1. American Psychiatric Association's draft guidelines for schizophrenia (December 2019; final version expected to be released in the summer of 2020)

2. A consensus opinion from a team of experts (Caroff et al., 2020)

Screening at baseline

1. Clinically assess all patients being started on an antipsychotic for the presence of any abnormal involuntary movements

2. If any involuntary movements are present, assess and quantify their severity using a structured instrument (e.g., AIMS)

Screening during follow up

We recommend instituting both steps 1 and 2 below for all patients receiving maintenance antipsychotic treatment.

1. At each visit, clinically assess patients for the presence of any abnormal involuntary movements.

This clinical assessment should consist of both of the following:

a. Asking the patient (and caregiver if present)

− Has the patient (or caregiver) noticed any current or recent abnormal movements?

b. Brief clinical examination to detect any abnormal involuntary movements

Although the APA practice guideline does not define clinical examination, the following two approaches have been suggested (Caroff et al., 2020):

− An informal clinical examination, simply observing for involuntary movements in the psychomotor component of the mental status exam.

− A semi-structured evaluation including selected tasks from the AIMS, e.g., opening mouth, rapid alternating hand movements.

2. At pre-scheduled timepoints, assess patients using a longer structured standardized instrument like the AIMS.

a. For patients at high risk (e.g., elderly, on first-generation antipsychotics), perform the AIMS at least every 6 months.

b. For patients not at high risk, perform the AIMS at least every 12 months.

If involuntary movements are present

If new-onset involuntary movements are identified or pre-existing involuntary movements have worsened:

− Ask whether the movements are distressing, have affected the patient's functioning or quality of life, or have been noted to have changed over time.

− Assess the involuntary movements with a structured instrument (e.g.,

AIMS)

Which structured assessment tool should we use?

For evaluation every 6 to 12 months, in our opinion, using the AIMS makes more sense than the DISCUS because it is extremely well known and has a standardized examination procedure.

In the recommendations for screening discussed above, it was recommended that patients should be assessed more frequently if they are at higher risk. Who are these patients (American Psychiatric Association, 2020)? The 11 risk factors listed have been organized by us into four categories:

Demographic risk factors

1. Older than 55 years

2. Women

Comorbidities

1. With a mood disorder

2. With a substance use disorder

3. With intellectual disability

4. With central nervous system injury

Treatment factors

1. With high cumulative exposure to antipsychotic medications

2. With particularly high potency dopamine D2 receptor antagonists

Previous side effects

1. With a history of an acute dystonic reaction

2. With a history of clinically-significant parkinsonism

3. With a history of akathisia.

Here's a mnemonic to help us to remember these 11 risk factors:

1. Mom (i.e., an older female)

2. M.i.s.c. (the 4 comorbidities). "Misc" is an abbreviation for miscellaneous, right?

3. Two "high"'s (high cumulative exposure, high potency)

4. A history of any of the other 3 movement disorders caused by antipsychotics

Abnormal Involuntary Movement Scale

The Abnormal Involuntary Movement Scale (AIMS) is the most widely used scale for systematically examining a patient for abnormal involuntary movements (e.g., tardive dyskinesia). Clinicians need four things related to the AIMS, all of which are being provided in this article.

1. Understand the proper use of the AIMS

2. Obtain a copy of the scoring sheet where multiple administrations of the scale can be recorded on the same page.

3. Know how to do the full and proper examination process that must be done before scoring the AIMS.

4. Know how to correctly score the severity of involuntary movements on the AIMS — each item and global severity.

The aims of the AIMS

1. Screening persons for the presence of involuntary movements, and

2. Assessing the severity of the involuntary movements if present.

Three commonly held fallacies about the AIMS

1. That AIMS only looks for choreoathetoid movements

Actually, the AIMS examination assesses a variety of involuntary movements. However, tremors should specifically be ignored while doing ratings on the AIMS.

2. That choreoathetoid movements noted on the AIMS examination are invariably those of tardive dyskinesia

There are other causes of choreoathetoid movements besides tardive dyskinesia, so all we can say is that the movements are consistent with TD.

3. That doing a formal AIMS examination is not essential

a) Many clinicians believe that they would identify tardive dyskinesia if present. However, one study found that the number of cases of tardive dyskinesia identified increased significantly after use of the AIMS was introduced (Munetz and Schulz, 1986).

b) Similarly, asking patients whether they have noted any involuntary movements is not sufficient. About half of persons with tardive dyskinesia deny being aware of any involuntary movements. Therefore, asking patients whether they have noted any involuntary movements is not an adequate way of assessing patients for possible tardive dyskinesia.

c) Legally, it would look quite bad if a person developed tardive dyskinesia and there was no documentation of systematic examinations on the chart. The implication would be that the person was not being carefully monitored for possible tardive dyskinesia.

How often should the AIMS examination be done?

1. At baseline

Since involuntary movements, including tardive dyskinesia, may be present even before any medication is taken, doing the AIMS examination at baseline is very important.

2. Twice a year

In addition, the AIMS examination should be done twice a year even if no involuntary movements have been noted.

3. More often under certain circumstances

a) If involuntary movements are detected

b) If the antipsychotic is changed, especially from a second-generation antipsychotic to a first-generation antipsychotic

c) If the antipsychotic is stopped (because tardive dyskinesia is suppressed by antipsychotics and may be first noticed after the antipsychotic is stopped).

d) If the antipsychotic dose is reduced (for the same reason as above)

The AIMS scoring sheet

The AIMS is not copyrighted and may be used freely. Rather than using one form per AIMS examination, it is better to use a scoring sheet that allows multiple administrations to be recorded on the same sheet. This allows for easy comparison with previous examinations.

ABNORMAL INVOLUNTARY MOVEMENT SCALE (AIMS)

Patient name:

Date					
Facial and Oral Movements	**1. Muscles of Facial Expression** e.g. movements of forehead, eyebrows periorbital area, cheeks, including frowning blinking, smiling, grimacing	0 1 2 3 4	0 1 2 3 4	0 1 2 3 4	0 1 2 3 4
	2. Lips and Perioral Area e.g., puckering, pouting, smacking	0 1 2 3 4	0 1 2 3 4	0 1 2 3 4	0 1 2 3 4
	3. Jaw e.g. biting, clenching, chewing, mouth opening, lateral movement	0 1 2 3 4	0 1 2 3 4	0 1 2 3 4	0 1 2 3 4
	4. Tongue Rate only increases in movement both in and out of mouth. NOT inability to sustain movement. Darting in and out of mouth.	0 1 2 3 4	0 1 2 3 4	0 1 2 3 4	0 1 2 3 4
Extremity Movements	**5. Upper (arms, wrists,, hands, fingers)** Include choreic movements (i.e., rapid, objectively purposeless, irregular, spontaneous) athetoid movements (i.e., slow, irregular, complex, serpentine). **Do not include tremor** (i.e., repetitive, regular, rhythmic)	0 1 2 3 4	0 1 2 3 4	0 1 2 3 4	0 1 2 3 4
	6. Lower (legs, knees, ankles, toes) e.g., lateral knee movement, foot tapping, heel dropping, foot squirming, inversion and eversion of foot.	0 1 2 3 4	0 1 2 3 4	0 1 2 3 4	0 1 2 3 4
Trunk Movements	**7. Neck, shoulders, hips** e.g., rocking, twisting, squirming, pelvic gyrations	0 1 2 3 4	0 1 2 3 4	0 1 2 3 4	0 1 2 3 4
Global	**8. Overall severity of abnormal**	0 1 2 3 4	0 1 2 3 4	0 1 2 3 4	0 1 2 3 4

261

Judgments	movements				
	9. Incapacitation due to abnormal movements	0 1 2 3 4	0 1 2 3 4	0 1 2 3 4	0 1 2 3 4
	10. Patient's awareness of abnormal movements. Rate only patient's report No awareness 0 Aware, no distress 1 Aware, mild distress 2 Aware, moderate distress 3 Aware, severe distress 4	0 1 2 3 4	0 1 2 3 4	0 1 2 3 4	0 1 2 3 4
Dental Status	11. Current problems with teeth and/or dentures	No Yes	No Yes	No Yes	No Yes
	12. Are dentures usually worn?	No Yes	No Yes	No Yes	No Yes
	13. Edentia?	No Yes	No Yes	No Yes	No Yes
	14. Do movements disappear in sleep?	No Yes	No Yes	No Yes	No Yes

Abnormal Involuntary Movement Scale (AIMS): Examination procedure

In order to be able to properly identify involuntary movements that may be present and to correctly score such movements on the Abnormal Involuntary Movement Scale, it is essential that the proper examination procedure should be followed. The examination procedure described here has been modified from that described by Munetz and Benjamin (1988).

Part 1. Informal observation

1. Observe the person at rest when s/he does not know that s/he is being observed. This can be before or after the rest of the examination.

2. Watch the patient while walking (e.g., to the office). Walking often makes upper extremity and orofacial dyskinesias more obvious

Part 2. Sitting quietly

1. Ideally, have the person sit in a chair with a hard or firm seat and without any arms. When the chair has arms, this tends to mask involuntary movements of the upper extremities.

2. Ask the person to not talk while being examined for any involuntary movements.

3. Have the person sit in the chair, keep the legs slightly apart and feet flat on the floor, and to put his hands on his knees.

4. Wait for a few seconds and systematically look at seven areas of the body for any involuntary movements. If the person cannot keep his hands and feet still, this may be an early sign of tardive dyskinesia.

5. Look at the person's breathing pattern. Look for any unusual movements of the abdomen. Look for any grunting, gasping, or sighing that can indicate respiratory dyskinesias.

Part 3. Take shoes off

If possible, ask the person to remove his shoes and socks so that movements of the toes can be observed. In tardive dyskinesia, movements of the toes are twisting in nature in contrast to akathisia or anxiety where foot tapping is more likely to be present.

Part 4. Hands hanging

Ask the person to sit with the hands hanging between the legs. In the case of a female patient wearing a dress or a long skirt, ask the person to place the wrists on the knees and leave the hands hanging over the knees.Systematically look at seven areas of the body for any involuntary movements. But, in particular, look for movements of the fingers.

Part 5. The mouth and tongue

1. Ask the person to open his mouth and observe the tongue at rest.

In my experience, when asked to open their mouth, people often protrude the tongue without being asked to do so. So, I say, "Please open your mouth. Keep your tongue in." Then ask the person to close his mouth. Repeat opening the mouth.

2. Ask the person to stick out his tongue. Then ask the person to put his tongue back in. Repeat sticking the tongue out.

Movements of the tongue can also be rated with the mouth closed by observing movements of the larynx (Lane et al., 1985).

Part 6. Activation procedure: Tapping the fingers

Ask the person to tap his thumb with each finger, one at a time, for about 10 to 15 seconds per finger. Do this first with one hand and then with the other. Finger tapping is an activating maneuver. Therefore, when the person is doing this, look not at the hands, but at other parts of the body because tapping the fingers may unmask dyskinesias in other parts of the body. In particular, look at the face and lower extremities because finger tapping is most likely to unmask dyskinesias in those parts.

Note: Sometimes, movements of fingers of the opposite hand occur while tapping the fingers of one hand. It is not clear what to do with this. Some authorities (e.g., Munetz et al., 1988) recommend that these contralateral movements should be ignored. Others (e.g., Lane et al., 1985) recommend that they should be rated but at one severity point below what they would be rated at normally. I don't agree with either of these views. In my independent opinion, it depends if the movements of the opposite hand are of the typical choreoathetoid type, they should be rated normally and treated as movements that emerged upon activation. If they are not choreoathetoid, they should be ignored because of that and not because they appeared on activation.

Part 7. Stand up

1. Ask the person to stand up. Look especially at the trunk. Truncal movements may be noted for the first time when the person stands up.

2. Ask the person to turn sideways so that you can observe the trunk (and other parts) in profile.

Part 8. Activation procedure: Extend arms out

Ask the person to extend both arms out with palms down. This is another activating measure. Look especially at the trunk, mouth, and legs.

Part 9. Activation procedure: Walk

1. Ask the person to walk a few steps, turn around, and walk back. Tell the person to, "Just relax and walk normally." This is the third and last activating measure. It is one of the most important parts of the examination in AIMS because involuntary movements of the fingers, hands, and arms

are most commonly revealed during this part of the examination.

However, unfortunately, this part of the examination is usually neglected in doing the AIMS. It is important that there be enough space for the person to walk several steps. Look at the hands and arms in addition to the gait.

2. Repeat—ask the person to again walk a few steps and then walk back.

What to do if any involuntary movements are noted

1. If chewing or similar movements are observed, ask the person if there is anything in his mouth (gum/candy) even if you did not obviously note that there was. If there is, ask him to remove it.

2. If any perioral movements are noted, ask the person if he has any loose teeth, dentures, or painful teeth.

3. If any involuntary movements are noted, ask the person if he has noted any involuntary movements anywhere in the body. About half of patients with tardive dyskinesia deny any awareness of abnormal movements.

4. If the person has noted involuntary movements, ask to what extent they a) bother him, and b) interfere with his activities. Surprisingly, many persons with tardive dyskinesia deny being bothered by involuntary movements.

Examination for Parkinsonism

Also, even though this is not a part of the AIMS examination per se, as part of the clinical evaluation, we should examine the person for parkinsonism as well. I don't agree with some sources who state that parkinsonian rigidity should also be noted on the AIMS scoring sheet; it is not an involuntary movement. While some sources have correctly noted that parkinsonian rigidity may mask tardive dyskinesia because the person's movements are diminished, I think the rigidity would have to be quite severe to prevent involuntary movements.

Abnormal Involuntary Movement Scale (AIMS): Scoring

Here are the detailed guidelines for rating involuntary movements seen on the Abnormal Involuntary Movement Scales (AIMS).

What to rate

1. Which types of movements?

Some sources, including the classic paper by Munetz and Benjamin (1988) suggest that all involuntary movements that are seen, except tremors, should be rated. However, the purpose of the AIMS is to identify and monitor tardive dyskinesia. On the other hand, it is hard to be certain that choreoathetoid movements seen during the AIMS examination are tardive dyskinesia or that they are medication-induced. Therefore, I recommend that only choreoathetoid movements consistent with tardive dyskinesia should be rated on the AIMS. While doing say, we should realize that these choreoathetoid movements may or may not be due to medication-induced tardive dyskinesia.

2. Which parts of the body?

Involuntary movements in seven different parts are rated:

— four are Facial/Oral (Muscles of Facial Expression, Lips and Perioral Area, Jaw, Tongue),

— two are Extremities (Upper, Lower), and

— one is the Trunk. The Trunk includes the "Neck, Shoulders, and Hips" as a single item.

Since "Lips and Perioral Area" is a separate category, for AIMS ratings, the category of "Muscles of Facial Expression" refers only to the forehead, eyebrows, periorbital area, and cheeks.

3. Examples of movements of different parts

Movements of the Muscles of Facial Expression include frowning, blinking, smiling, grimacing, etc.

Movements of the Lips and Perioral Area include puckering pouting, smacking, etc.

Movements of the Jaw include biting, clenching, chewing, mouth opening, lateral movement of the lower jaw, etc.

Movements of the Lower extremity include lateral knee movement, foot tapping, heel dropping, foot squirming,and inversion and eversion of the foot.

Movements of the Trunk (neck, shoulder, hips) include rocking, twisting, squirming, pelvic gyrations, etc.

Rating the severity of movements

1. The rating of severity of involuntary movements in each of the seven parts is done on a five point scale:

0 Absent

1 Minimal (may be extreme normal)

2 Mild

3 Moderate

4 Severe.

Caution! We should not use a rating of 1 for mild movements. A rating of 1 should be used only for movements that are so minimal that they may, in fact, be normal.

The problem, of course, is that it is not specified what Mild, Moderate, and Severe mean. It's largely a matter of judgment.

2. The severity should be rated based on the quality, frequency, and amplitude of the involuntary movement.

3. Rate the highest severity of movement observed at any time during the examination. So if while the AIMS examination is being done, if movements of a particular part are mild at one time but severe during another time, do not average out the severity. Rather, rate that part of the body as having the highest severity of movements observed.

4. The original instructions for scoring the AIMS noted that movements occurring only on activation should be scored one point lower than those seen without activation. However, most subsequent experts don't

recommend following this convention. They give the following two reasons (Munetz and Benjamin, 1988):

a) There is no actual evidence that involuntary movements seen only on activation have less clinical significance than those that are seen spontaneously.

b) And this one is the more convincing reason for me—the activating measures used in the AIMS examination are similar to movements a person makes in the course of day-to-day activities. So if the movements are showing up during the activation procedures, they are probably showing up in the person's day-to-day life as well.

Therefore, I too recommend that we not rate movements seen only on activation as less severe than those seen spontaneously

Instructions regarding rating specific body parts

1. For movements of the tongue, one helpful way to know which movements to rate is to rate only movements of the tongue that are increased both inside and outside the mouth.

2. If involuntary movements of the tongue cause it to go between the upper and lower teeth in any direction, forward or sideways, this should be rated as at least moderate severity (i.e., a rating of 3).

3. If movements of the tongue or jaw lead to movement of the lips, this should not be considered to be an involuntary movement of the lips.

4. However, if both upper and lower lips move, this should not be attributed simply to movement of the jaw since movement of the lower jaw should not lead to movement of the upper lip.

5. Sometimes, movements of fingers of the opposite hand occurs while tapping the fingers of one hand. It is not clear what to do with this. Some authorities (e.g., Muntez et al., 1988) recommend that these contralateral movements should be ignored. Others (e.g., Lane et al., 1985) recommend that they should be rated but at one severity point below what they would be rated at normally. I don't agree with either of these views. In my independent opinion, it depends if the movements of the opposite hand are of the typical choreoathetoid type, they should be rated normally and treated as movements that emerged upon activation. If they are not choreoathetoid, they should be ignored because of that and not because

they appeared on activation.

Global score

After the severity of involuntary movements in each area is scored, it is time to assign a Global score for the severity of involuntary movements in this person.

1. By convention, the Global score is the highest score in any of the seven body parts examined.

2. However, an alternative way is to add the scores from the seven parts.

Optional ratings

After this, there are some ratings on the AIMS that are not really part of the examination or necessary. I personally would be OK with skipping them during a busy clinical visit.

1. Incapacitation due to the involuntary movements. On examination, how are we supposed to know that? A person can have clear-cut perioral movements but not be incapacitated in the sense that he can still speak or eat. The involuntary movements have to be quite severe before bodily functions are directly impaired.

2. Awareness of the abnormal movements. Not something that can be examined, of course; we have to ask the patient. This is not a measure of the severity of movements but includes a rating of the distress. I think that awareness does not automatically relate to distress. I wish they that the item was called distress and had the option to rate it as "N/A Unaware" apart from 0 = no distress.

3. Problems with teeth or wearing dentures. This is only relevant if perioral or jaw movements are noted and can be skipped if such movements are not present. While the instructions don't explicitly state this, it is implied that perioral or jaw movements should be rated as observed even if you think they are due to the problems with the teeth or due to the presence of dentures. I don't think this should be an item on the AIMS. It is simply part of the examination procedure to take into account.

Management of tardive dyskinesia: First-line options

Regular screening for tardive dyskinesia and early detection are by far the most things we can do to manage the risk of tardive dyskinesia in patients who are on an antipsychotic.

If TD does occur, here are the steps that we should systematically consider:

1. Taper off anticholinergic medications

Anticholinergic medications may make TD worse and should, therefore, be tapered off (Egan et al. 1997).

2. Stop the causative dopamine-blocking medication if possible

While this may improve the TD only in a small minority of patients, presumably it will reduce the risk of further progression of the TD.

However, it is important to not panic and suddenly stop the medication. Suddenly stopping the medication may cause the existing TD symptoms to worsen or lead to withdrawal dyskinesia that was not noted earlier.

And there is another problem. Dopamine-blocking medications reduce symptoms of TD in the short run, but may worsen them in the long-run. We should be aware of this trade off and not be tempted to routinely suppress the symptoms of TD by increasing the antipsychotic dose.

3. Switch to a second-generation antipsychotic

Since second-generation antipsychotics appear to have a lower risk of TD, if the patient is on a first-generation antipsychotic, it may seem appropriate to switch to a second-generation antipsychotic.

A review by the American Academy of Neurology (Bhidayasiri et al., 2013) concluded that data are insufficient to either support or refute the efficacy of this strategy. However, the CATIE study, an important, large study of antipsychotic treatment in persons with schizophrenia, provides support for recommending switching to a second-generation antipsychotic. Many of the participants had TD at the start of the study. Of these, those who were randomized to receive a second-generation antipsychotic showed a significant decrease in the severity of TD (Caroff et al., 2011).

4. Switch to quetiapine

A one-year randomized, controlled clinical trial found treatment with quetiapine to be superior to haloperidol for the treatment of TD (Emsley et al., 2004). The mean dose of quetiapine was 400 mg/day. At 12 months, 55% of persons treated with quetiapine had shown 50% or greater reduction in severity of TD compared to 28% of those treated with haloperidol. That's a 27% difference in response which would be considered clinically very useful.

5. Consider a VMAT2 inhibitor if it is available and economically possible

When VMAT2 is inhibited, this reduces the transport of dopamine and other monoamine neurotransmitters into vesicles where they would be protected from degradation by monoamine oxidase. So, gradually, the dopamine gets depleted. This leads to improvement in TD.

As of October 2020, three VMAT2 inhibitors are available (alphabetically): deutetrabenazine, tetrabenazine, and valbenazine. Of these, as of August 2017, only valbenazine is FDA-approved for the treatment of TD, but the other two also have data supporting their use.

Unfortunately, all three of these medications are very expensive, especially valbenazine and deutetrabenazine that were more recently introduced.

How well does valbenazine work for TD? A 50% or greater reduction in the AIMS score was defined as a "response". Using this definition, 40% of persons who received valbenazine were responders compared with 9% of those on placebo. That is a 31% difference in the response rates on drug versus placebo, which is clinically very significant.

Management of tardive dyskinesia: Second-line options

I consider the following options discussed below to be second-line for one of the three reasons:

— Because they may have other problems associated with their use

— Because the evidence-base is not as strong, or

– Because their benefits are only temporary.

1. Switch to clozapine

A small open-label study in patients with severe TD treated with clozapine and followed for several years have suggested that not only does clozapine have a low likelihood of causing TD, it seems to actually treat it (Louza and Bassitt, 2005). Of course, clozapine can have its own problems, so it can't be a first-line treatment for most patients. Agree?

2. Increase dopamine blockade

When there is a need to immediately control the TD movements–for example, if the patient is attending an important social event–temporarily increasing the dose of the antipsychotic will reduce the TD symptoms. In a randomized, controlled trial, risperidone 6 mg/day was efficacious for reducing the involuntary movements in many, but not all, persons with TD (Bai et al., 2003).

However, this is probably not a good strategy for most patients because in the long run increased exposure to antipsychotics increases the risk of persistence and worsening of the TD.

3. Consider adding a benzodiazepine for the short-term

While one guideline (Bhidayasiri et al., 2013) noted that clonazepam probably improves TD and should be considered as a treatment option, a review with by the Cochrane Collaboration concluded that the data are contradictory on whether or not benzodiazepines can reduce TD and that use of benzodiazepines should be considered experimental (Bhoopathi and Soares-Weiser, 2006).

In a small, randomized, controlled clinical trial in which clonazepam produced partial improvement in TD symptoms, patients with predominantly dystonic symptoms showed greater benefit than patients with predominantly choreoathetoid dyskinesias (Thaker et al., 1990). Relatively high doses of clonazepam will probably be needed.

In a blinded, flexible-dose study (Thaker et al., 1990), the dose of clonazepam used was 2 to 4.5 mg/day. Also, the effect of clonazepam tended to wear off after a few months (Thaker et al., 1990), so its use is recommended for up to about three months (Vijayakumar and Jancovic, 2016).

4. Consider adding amantadine for the short-term

There are two published randomized, controlled clinical trials supporting the use of amantadine for this purpose (Angus et al., 1997; Pappa et al., 2010). The American Academy of Neurology guideline supported its use as one option for the treatment of tardive syndromes (Bhidayasiri et al., 2006). So, we can consider amantadine as a second-line option. If it is used, the dose would start at 100 mg/day and should probably be increased at weekly intervals to 300 mg/day.

5. Consider adding Ginkgo biloba

The American Academy of Neurology guideline notes that Ginkgo biloba probably improves tardive syndrome and should be considered a treatment option (Bhidayasiri et al., 2006). There are at least three studies from China that found Ginkgo biloba to be efficacious for the treatment of TD (Zheng et al., 2016). In one of them (Zhang et al., 2011), about half of the patients responded to treatment with Ginkgo biloba extract. So, we could consider Ginkgo biloba as a second-line option for the treatment of tardive dyskinesia.

Comparing the VMAT2 inhibitors

Three medications that are VMAT2 inhibitors are available in the US. All three of these medications are "selective" VMAT2 inhibitors. Alphabetically, they are:

1. Deutetrabenazine (Austedo®)

Deutetetrabenazine (Austedo®) was developed by adding deuterium to tetrabenazine. This modifies the pharmacokinetic profile and leads to more uniform levels of the drug.

It has been shown to be efficacious for tardive dyskinesia (Anderson et al., 2017).

Deutetrabenazine (Austedo®) was approved by the FDA in 2017 for the treatment of chorea associated with Huntington's disease and later in 2017 for the treatment of tardive dyskinesia in adults.

2. Tetrabenazine (Xenazine®)

Tetrabenazine has been around for a while and is FDA-approved for the treatment of Huntington's disease. Even though it is now generic, it is still expensive–at least $1500 per month for thirty tablets of 25 mg (per goodrx.com).

3. Valbenazine (Ingrezza®)

This was the first medication to be FDA-approved (in April 2017) for the treatment of tardive dyskinesia.

Which VMAT-2 inhibitor should we choose?

1. Depression and suicidality

Especially for use in patients with mental health problems, it is important to note that both tetrabenazine and deutetrabenazine carry boxed ("black box") warnings that the medication "Increases the risk of depression and suicidal thoughts and behavior (suicidality) in patients with Huntington's disease." The boxed warning then makes recommendations for caution and monitoring and ends by stating that tetrabenazine/deutetrabenazine is "contraindicated in patients who are suicidal, and in patients with untreated or inadequately treated depression."

In the valbenazine studies, no increased risk of depression or suicidality was found. Therefore, valbenazine (Ingrezza) does not carry any warning about possible depression or suicidality. A major reason for this difference may be that the valbenazine studies are in tardive dyskinesia and the tetrabenazine and deutetrabenazine studies are in Huntington's disease. Persons with Huntington's disease are very prone to developing depression and suicidal ideation. So, even with valbenazine, it will be wise for us to still be cautious, especially if using it in persons at higher risk of depression or suicidality.

Also, persons who were at higher risk of suicidal behaviors were excluded from participation in these studies. So, for the first few years, it will be wise for us to still be cautious with all of these medications.

(Note: Valbenazine does carry warnings about the risk of somnolence and of QT prolongation in high-risk patients.)

Because tetrabenazine is generic, we may wrongly think that it is cheap. According to goodrx.com (checked in September, 2020), thirty 25 mg tablets of tetrabenazine cost $395 or more. While tetrabenazine has been available for many years, it has been nearly impossible to get insurance companies to pay for it.

The manufacturers of valbenazine (Ingrezza®) and deutetrabenazine (Austedo®) have online programs to help prescribing clinicians and patients get the medication approved. The FDA approval of these medications for tardive dyskinesia has made it a bit more likely that insurances will pay for these medications despite their high cost.

Valbenazine (Ingrezza®) and VMAT2

Valbenazine (Ingrezza®) is a selective inhibitor of vesicular monoamine transporter 2 (VMAT 2), that is FDA-approved for the treatment of adults with tardive dyskinesia. It is the first medication ever to be FDA-approved for the treatment of tardive dyskinesia. However, it is not the first or only VMAT 2 inhibitor. Nor is it the first or only medication to be shown to be effective for tardive dyskinesia.

What is VMAT 2?

VMAT2 sounds like the name of a rocket, I know. But actually, the vesicular monoamine transporter 2 (VMAT2) is a protein in presynaptic neurons that release monoamine neurotransmitters like dopamine. In the presynaptic neuron, VMAT2 transports these monoamines from the cytoplasm into synaptic vesicles. Once in the synaptic vesicles, the monoamines are protected from being metabolized by monoamine oxidase.

When VMAT 2 is inhibited, as with valbenazine treatment, uptake of monoamines (like dopamine) into synaptic vesicles is reduced. Therefore, the monoamines are not protected within vesicles and get metabolized. The gradual depletion of dopamine is, presumably, what leads to improvement in the tardive dyskinesia.

The "2" does not mean it is an improved version of VMAT! VMAT occurs in two forms: VMAT 1 that is found in the periphery and VMAT2 that is found in the central nervous system.

The term "selective" VMAT2 inhibitor means that the medication inhibits only VMAT2 and not VMAT1. And that it does not have any other pharmacological effects, e.g., on various postsynaptic receptors.

Does vitamin E work for tardive dyskinesia

Antioxidants such as vitamin E have been tried for treating tardive dyskinesia. Why antioxidants? Because of a hypothesis that the use of dopamine receptor blocking drugs leads to the production of free radicals that are toxic to the brain and are involved in the pathophysiology of tardive dyskinesia (Cadet and Kahler, 1994; Cadet and Lohr, 1989). It was speculated that antioxidant medications, like vitamin E, by neutralizing the free radicals produced by the use of dopamine receptor blocking drugs may be helpful in preventing or even treating tardive dyskinesia.

Does vitamin E work for tardive dyskinesia?

The answer to this question is: Yes and No. Read on and you will see why I say that.

In 2018, the Cochrane Collaboration (a highly respected group that systematically combines the results of randomized, controlled, clinical trials) updated its report on the use of vitamin E for tardive dyskinesia (Soares-Weiser et al., 2018). Here is what it found:

– 13 randomized, controlled clinical trials with a total of 478 participants

– The participants were adults with schizophrenia or another chronic psychiatric disorder who had developed tardive dyskinesia while on an antipsychotic medication.

– Vitamin E was not more efficacious than placebo for the treatment of tardive dyskinesia (Soares-Weiser et al., 2018).

[A subsequent meta-analysis that included two more clinical trials (Artukoglu et al., 2020) found vitamin E to be more efficacious than placebo even for reducing the symptoms of tardive dyskinesia. But, it acknowledged that, due to certain issues with the research, this effectiveness is probably overstated.]

– But, those treated with vitamin E had much less risk of a further worsening of the tardive dyskinesia than those treated with placebo (Soares-Weiser et al., 2018). A word of caution—the total number of patients in studies that evaluated this was small, so this needs confirmation.

Any supporting evidence?

Animal studies can be helpful as a supplement to the much more important human data.

In an animal model of tardive dyskinesia, rats who received vitamin E developed fewer involuntary chewing movements (e.g., An et al., 2016; Shi et al., 2016).

Bottom line

The following conclusions and comments (as of July 2020) are based on my own understanding of the literature and my consultations with several leading experts in the field.

1. There is no convincing evidence that vitamin E reduces antipsychotic-induced tardive dyskinesia.

2. But, it may reduce further worsening of tardive dyskinesia. This finding does not appear surprising if we go back to the hypothesis about how vitamin E may work for tardive dyskinesia. If it is true and vitamin E works as an antioxidant neutralizing toxic free radicals, one might expect it to reduce further damage in patients who are continuing to take an antipsychotic.

We may hypothesize that vitamin E may be more helpful against the progression of tardive dyskinesia if the TD is mild and of shorter duration. I hope that further studies are soon conducted to evaluate whether vitamin E may reduce the further progression of tardive dyskinesia, especially if it is introduced early on.

Unfortunately, in the Cochrane Collaboration's meta-analysis (Soares-Weiser et al., 2019), it was not possible to evaluate whether the effect of vitamin E for tardive dyskinesia was different depending on the duration of tardive dyskinesia because none of the studies reported data separately based on the duration of the tardive dyskinesia.

If the hypothesis that vitamin E may be helpful in reducing further progression mainly if the tardive dyskinesia is mild and of shorter duration is true, then this is another reason to emphasize regular and careful monitoring of all patients treated with an antipsychotic for the development of tardive dyskinesia.

3. To anticipate a question that may arise, we don't know whether taking vitamin E along with a dopamine receptor blocking drug (especially a first-generation antipsychotic) before tardive dyskinesia even develops might reduce the incidence or severity of tardive dyskinesia.

4. Another thing to note is that vitamin E is of two broad types: tocopherols and tocotrienols (Abraham et al., 2019). Clinical trials have typically used alpha-tocopherol but tocotrienols are more potent as anti-oxidants. I would like to see future studies of vitamin E for tardive dyskinesia that use tocotrienols rather than tocopherols.

What dose of vitamin E?

It is not entirely clear what the optimal dose of vitamin E may be (Artukoglu et al., 2020). But, if a clinician and patient decide to use vitamin E to try to reduce further worsening of tardive dyskinesia, a dose of 1200 to 1600 IU per day was suggested (Aia et al., 2011). All but one of the studies included in the Cochrane Collaboration's meta-analysis (Soares-Weiser et al., 2018) used 1200 to 1600 IU per day of vitamin E.

The total dose should be given in three divided doses per day.

But, wait! Are these doses of vitamin E safe?

Vitamin E: A primer for clinicians

How much vitamin E do we need?

The Recommended Dietary Allowance (RDA) of vitamin E for adults is 15 mg/day, though there is considerable uncertainty as to whether this estimate is correct (NIH Office of Dietary Supplements).

Note: The FDA has mandated changes in product labeling from IUs to mg. Conversion between IUs and mg is as follows (NIH Office of Dietary Supplements):

1 IU of the synthetic form is equivalent to 0.45 mg of alpha-tocopherol.

Several national surveys have found that most persons in the USA take less than the Recommended Dietary Allowance of vitamin E though, due to uncertainty about the amounts of cooking oil used, the surveys may have underestimated how much vitamin E was in the diet of respondents (NIH Office of Dietary Supplements). This is particularly a concern for persons taking a low-fat diet because cooking oils contain significant quantities of vitamin E.

Good dietary sources of vitamin E

Some of the best dietary sources of vitamin E are:

1. Various cooking oils

2. Seeds and nuts

3. Green leafy vegetables

Here are some examples of the vitamin E content of these foods:

Sunflower seeds, 1 ounce (dry, roasted): 7.5 mg (half of the RDA for adults)

Almonds 1 ounce (dry, roasted): 7 mg

Peanut butter, 2 tablespoons: 3 mg

Peanuts, 1 ounce (dry, roasted): 2 mg
Vitamin E in commonly used multivitamins

The amount of vitamin E (in mg) contained in some common multivitamin brands in the US is close to the RDA of 15 mg per day:

Centrum Adults®: 13.5 mg

Kirkland Signature Daily Multi®: 13.5 mg

One-a-Day Men's Health Formula® (the brand that I take): 10 mg

One-a-Day Women's Formula®: 7.5 mg

Vitamin E: Potential adverse effects and drug interactions

Many people take various vitamin, mineral, and other supplements without any concern for their possible adverse effects and for drug interactions between these supplements and the medications they are taking.

Also, the dose of vitamin E that has been used in tardive dyskinesia studies 1200 to 1600 IU per day, is equivalent to 540 to 720 mg/day. So, this dose is massive compared to the Recommended Dietary Allowance of 15 mg/day! We have to be concerned about whether this is safe.

Potential adverse effects and other safety concerns

1. At the doses being recommended, gastrointestinal side effects (nausea, diarrhea, flatulence, etc) can occur.

2. Several meta-analyses of studies have found that a higher intake of vitamin E is associated with a lower risk of various cancers (e.g., Lin et al., 2019; Cui et al., 2018; Zhu et al., 2017). But, the data are not consistent. In part, this may be because persons with some genetic polymorphisms may be more likely to have a cancer-lowering effect from vitamin E (e.g., Hall et al., 2019). So, whether and in what situations vitamin E may reduce the risk of some cancers remains uncertain.

Also, we should know that one large study shocked the scientific community when, instead of a reduction in the risk of prostate cancer, a slightly increased risk of prostate cancer was found in persons given vitamin E (Klein et al., 2011). So, vitamin E, especially at very high doses, cannot be assumed to be benign.

3. There is a small amount of data that huge doses of vitamin E (e.g., 400 mg/day) may impair the effectiveness of tamoxifen in women with breast cancer (Podszun and Frank, 2014).

4. Huge doses of vitamin E may also appear to reduce the serum levels of cyclosporine A, which is used to prevent organ transplant rejection (Podszun and Frank, 2014).

5. High doses of vitamin E should not be given to persons taking aspirin or warfarin. Megadoses of vitamin E may impair platelet aggregation and interfere with the metabolism of vitamin K. This may increase the risk of abnormal bleeding when given along with other medications that impair hemostasis.

Note: At modest doses, vitamin E does not appear to cause clinically significant drug interactions (Podszun and Frank, 2014).

Is antipsychotic-induced tardive dyskinesia reversible if the antipsychotic is stopped?

In patients starting an antipsychotic medication that they may take for many months or years, tardive dyskinesia (TD) is one of the most important concerns for patients, their loved ones, and the treating clinicians. Often clinicians say to the patient something like—"We'll regularly monitor you for these involuntary movements and if they occur, we can always stop the antipsychotic."

A 2019 review article (Ricciardi et al., 2019) also recommended: "The first-line management of tardive dyskinesia is the withdrawal of antipsychotic medication if clinically feasible." We hear this recommendation often, but is it based on facts?

Informed consent?

We know that in the short term tardive dyskinesia may paradoxically worsen on stopping the antipsychotic. But, a crucial question to answer as part of the informed consent process is: If we are able to stop all antipsychotic treatment (which is often at least an option in patients with mood disorders), will the involuntary movements eventually subside?

In other words, is early tardive dyskinesia reversible in most cases?

OR, are we misleading the patient by implying, even indirectly, that if the antipsychotic is stopped early enough, the TD is likely to improve or even resolve completely?

Practice Guidelines

The American Academy of Neurology's practice guideline on the treatment of tardive syndrome (Bhidayasiri et al., 2013 and 2018) explicitly asked this question—Is withdrawal of dopamine receptor blocking agents an effective treatment for tardive syndromes? It concluded that "Data are insufficient to support or refute" this.

The draft American Psychiatric Association practice guideline on the treatment of schizophrenia, unpublished as of July 2019, does not say anything about the question we are discussing.

Let's look elsewhere to see what information we can find to help us answer the question of whether or not tardive dyskinesia is often reversible if all antipsychotic treatment can be stopped.

Meta-analysis of studies

The conclusion of the Cochrane Collaboration's review (Bergman et al., 2018) is similar to that of the American Academy of Neurology's practice guideline. It states in its "Plain Language Summary:"

"It is not known if strategies such as dose reduction, 'drug holidays', and stopping medication are helpful in the treatment of tardive dyskinesia."

Small studies

The report of the American Psychiatric Association Task Force on tardive dyskinesia (American Psychiatric Association, 1992) reviewed a few small studies. Let's see, briefly, what some of these studies found.

Jeste et al. (1979): 21 patients, antipsychotic stopped for three months, TD resolved in 12 patients (a little more than half of the patients). Importantly, the patients in whom the TD did not resolve even after stopping the antipsychotic had:

– A longer duration of treatment with antipsychotics

– More (sic) periods of being free of antipsychotics for two months or more.

The authors warned that we should not try to give patients "drug holidays" thinking that it will reduce the chances of developing tardive dyskinesia.

Klawans et al. (1984): 5 patients who were off antipsychotics for 2.5 to 5 years and in whom the TD did not resolve in the first few months but did resolve later on. The authors commented that we should not assume that even persistent TD is necessarily permanent.

Other authors also reported resolution of tardive dyskinesia in many, but not all, patients in whom the antipsychotic was stopped (Itoh and Yagi, 1979; Jeste and Wyatt, 1982; Fahn, 1985).

Bottom Line

There are no published randomized, controlled studies evaluating whether or not TD is reversible on stopping the antipsychotic.

But, that does not mean that we have nothing whatsoever to say to our patients during the informed consent process. From the limited, non-randomized data that we do have, we find that the cup is half full (or half empty, if you prefer to look at it that way).

The good news is that:

1. If antipsychotic treatment is stopped for several months, tardive dyskinesia may be reversible in many patients. Maybe about half of them.

2. In some others, the dyskinetic movements may even eventually subside after having persisted for two years or more.

On the other hand, we must be honest in admitting that even if the antipsychotic is stopped when the tardive dyskinesia is identified, the movements may persist in many patients.

Let's admit it—it is difficult to say to patients right as we are recommending starting an antipsychotic that if you develop TD, EVEN IF we stop all antipsychotic treatment, the TD may not be reversible. But, doesn't informed consent mean being able to tell the patient not just the good news but the not-so-good news as well?

TREMORS

Medication-induced tremors: An overview

Tremor is the commonest movement disorder caused by psychotropic medications. While physicians frequently do not consider it to be a particularly important adverse effect, patients find it embarrassing and quite distressing. Not surprisingly, therefore, tremors are one of the leading causes of discontinuation of medications — for example, discontinuation of mood stabilizers by patients with bipolar disorder.

Important tip: Do NOT consider tremor to be a minor side effect. Patients may "vote with their feet" by stopping the medication.

Etiology of tremors

"Physiological" tremors (a benign tremor that may be present in normal persons) are postural and in parkinsonism, the tremor can be postural in addition to being classically a resting tremor. Physiological tremors are usually hard to see. However, they may become more noticeable when the person is tired or under stress, or in medical conditions like fever, hyperthyroidism, drug withdrawal, etc.

Essential tremors are the most common movement disorder. They generally start gradually and slowly progress. Flexion-extension movement of the wrist is typical. Movement of the head front and back or side-to-side may also occur. A family history of essential tremor is present in the great majority of cases.

Medications commonly associated with tremors and the incidences of tremor with them are shown in the table below. (N/A denotes that the tremor was not a treatment-emergent adverse event that occurred in at least 1% of subjects in clinical trials and twice as often as on placebo, which is the definition of "adverse effect" I use.)

Category	Medication	Incidence of tremor
Mood stabilizers	Lithium	Common but exact incidence unclear
	Divalproex sodium	25%
	Lamotrigine	4%
Antidepressants	SSRIs	8%

	Bupropion	21%
	Vilazodone	2%
	Vortioxetine	N/A
Antipsychotics	Aripiprazole	6%
	Olanzapine	6%
	Quetiapine	2%
	Ziprasidone	N/A
Other	Buspirone	1%

With antidepressants, tremors also can occur during antidepressant discontinuation. When medications are used in combination, the incidence of tremor is generally higher. As always, such a situation should prompt a reassessment of the risk-benefit ratio in collaboration with the patient.

Alcohol and benzodiazepines tend to diminish many kinds of tremors, though not usually tremors associated with Parkinson's disease.

Factors that make the tremor better or worse

Medication-induced tremor is more common in older patients. It tends to occur early in treatment and may diminish in some patients. However, if the person continues on the medication, it tends to get worse as the person ages.

Management of medication-induced tremor

When a tremor is clearly troublesome, if possible the causative drug should be stopped or the dose reduced. However, in practice this is easier said than done.

Coffee can worsen many types of tremors and its use should therefore be minimized. In the case of lithium-induced tremor, it should be kept in mind that caffeine increases excretion of lithium. Therefore, if caffeine is reduced, the dose of lithium may need to be adjusted, otherwise the tremor may, in fact, worsen instead of improving.

Changing to a sustained-release preparation, if available, tends to reduce tremors by reducing the peak concentration.

Giving the medication as a single dose at bedtime, if feasible, may help because the peak concentration will occur while the person is asleep.

In general, medication-induced tremors tend to be dose related and, therefore, if dose reduction is feasible, it may reduce the tremors.

If this is possible, other medications (e.g., beta-2 agonists) that could be contributing to the tremor (in addition to the psychotropic medication) should also be stopped or reduced in dose.

Anticholinergics (e.g., benztropine 2-6 mg/day) or amantadine are quite helpful in the treatment of tremors associated with drug-induced Parkinsonism.

Beta blockers have been found to be useful not only for lithium-induced tremors but also for valproate-induced ones. For details about the management of lithium-induced tremors, see How to manage lithium-induced tremor

A variety of other drugs have been used in the treatment of tremors but these either have limited response rates or significant adverse effects. I suggest that if the measures discussed above fail most clinicians should probably obtain a consultation with a neurologist with expertise in movement disorders.

How to examine a person with tremors

Basic characteristics of the tremor

1. Fine or Coarse?

The first thing to do in evaluating a person with tremor is to see if the tremor is fine or coarse? By coarse, we mean that the amplitude of the movements is greater.

Tip: Fine tremors are harder to see. On examination, if a tremor is hard to see from a distance, have the patient spread his fingers and then put a sheet of paper on the outstretched hand. The tremor will now be better seen as vibration of the sheet of paper.

A benign lithium tremor is typically fine while one due to lithium toxicity is coarse. Tremors due to divalproex sodium are typically high frequency and low amplitude. Thus, these tremors are similar to benign essential tremors.

2. Unilateral or bilateral? If bilateral, symmetrical or asymmetrical?

Is it bilaterally symmetrical or is it either unilateral or asymmetrical? Medication-induced tremors tend to be symmetrical though tremors associated with drug–induced Parkinsonism are often asymmetrical.

Type of tremor

The next steps are to examine the tremor's association with posture and movement. While tremors can be classified in different ways, there are basically four different situations in which you can assess the tremor. The Movement Disorders Society classifies tremors into Resting, Postural, Simple kinetic or Action, and Intention tremors. This is based on when observing when the tremor is worse with relation to rest or movement.

A *resting tremor* is best seen when the body part is not being voluntarily used and is completely supported against gravity. It becomes less when that body part moves.

A *postural tremor* is best seen when the person is holding a posture, a state of static contraction.

A *simple kinetic or action tremor* is becomes more apparent when the patient moves to perform an action.

Lastly, an *intention tremor* is a tremor that worsens during the last part of a movement.

How to examine a tremor

1. Observe the tremor with the person sitting comfortably, with his hands resting comfortably in his lap, and when he does not think he is being observed. You can also facilitate observing the leg for a tremor by observing the person when the legs are crossed, i.e., on foot is not on the ground.

Tip: It is important and helpful to remember that the tremors of parkinsonism (due to Parkinson's disease or to a medication) are best seen at rest.

2. Have the person stretch his arms up horizontally in front of him and hold them in this position and observe for any tremor.

Important tip: Almost all drug-induced tremors are postural. (However, the tremor may persist in action or at rest.)

3. Observe the person for tremors during natural movement for the presence of Simple kinetic tremors that become more prominent during movement.

4. Ask the patient to stretch his arm out, extend his index finger, and then bring the arm back to touch his nose with the tip of the index finger. As the index finger approaches the nose, see if it shows clear worsening of the tremor, i.e., is an Intention tremor present.

Tip: An Intention tremor is classically found in cerebellar disease.

When I was recently examining a patient in this manner and explaining the process to a trainee, the patient remarked that the fact that his tremor was postural and not an action tremor must explain why his hands trembled when he was holding his golf club in position but not when he was swinging the golf club!

Ruling out other causes of tremors

Mental health clinicians are, of course, most interested in tremors caused by our medications. But, other causes of tremors must be ruled out.

1. Most importantly, the first thing to make sure is that the tremor is not a sign that the dose of the medication is too high. This can be done by seeing if the tremor has worsened with increased dose of the medication, checking the level of the medication, looking for other symptoms and signs of toxicity (other than the tremor), and so on.

2. Laboratory tests: For example, in any person who has a postural tremor, we must make sure to rule out hyperthyroidism.

3. Tip: In the history, it is important to see whether the tremor has worsened over time. A lack of gradual worsening of the tremor over time may suggest a medication-induced tremor rather than one that is caused by an underlying progressive neurological disease.

4. Tip: If needed, give the patient a task requiring concentration.

Tremors due to physical medical conditions tend to worsen when this is done while a tremor due to anxiety or other psychological reason tends to diminish.

How to monitor change in the severity of a tremor

It is useful to monitor the severity of tremors over time, including for assessing response to any intervention. Here are some ways in which you can monitor the progress:

1. Draw a neat spiral and ask the patient to copy it exactly (see figure below).

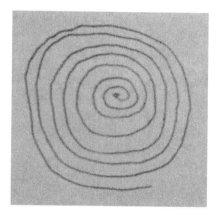

The tremor will be apparent in the irregularity of the line. At subsequent visits, you can have the patient copy the spiral again, allowing you to see if there is any change in the tremor.

2. Alternatively, have the patient write a standard piece of text (e.g., his name and address) on a blank sheet of paper, i.e., without any lines to help guide the handwriting. In most cases, the tremor is apparent in the writing. In subsequent visits, have the patient write the same text on a fresh sheet of blank paper, without looking at the previous sample of handwriting. By putting the two sheets of paper side by side, one can quite easily note whether the tremor has or has not improved.

3. Give the patient a cup of water and observe the tremor while the patient drinks the water.

4. Using my smartphone, I sometimes make a short film of the patient's hands (with outstretched arms). Since the patient's face is not filmed, only the hands, there is no real concern about privacy. The film can then be reviewed in the future to evaluate any change in the severity of the tremor.

Lithium-induced benign tremor

Why is lithium-induced tremor important?

There is something about tremors that make them particularly unacceptable to patients. In part, this may be because they are visible to others. Many patients have complained to me that it was embarrassing for them for others to notice that their hands were trembling—at work or in social situations.

When we think about why people stop lithium treatment, we may think it is due to serious problems like renal impairment, hypothyroidism, hyperparathyroidism, etc. But actually, the three commonest reasons why patients stop taking lithium are (in no particular order): tremors, weight gain, and cognitive impairment (Mago et al., 2014). Let's not ignore so-called "benign" tremors!

Also, lithium-induced tremors can either be benign or may indicate toxicity. We must be able to distinguish between the two.

So, it is important for clinicians who prescribe lithium to be able to identify, monitor, assess, and treat lithium-induced tremors.

What is the lithium-induced benign tremor like?

How common is it? The prevalence may depend on many factors, but overall about 27% of patients on lithium have a tremor (Gelenberg and Jefferson, 1995).

Location: It is typically present in the hands and is symmetrical.

Relation to posture: It is a postural tremor. That is, rather than at rest, it is most apparent if the person holds the arms and hands up against gravity. This means that it is quite apparent when the person is holding something like a cup up. It is likely to be prominent in actions like writing or pouring a liquid (Baek et al., 2014).

Amplitude: Almost always, a benign lithium-induced tremor is fine, that is, it has low amplitude. Fine tremors are not usually noticeable from a distance.

Appearance: It usually appears soon after lithium is started or the dose is increased. But sometimes it can appear later on.

Relation to lithium levels: Not only the tremor of lithium toxicity, but even the benign tremor tends to be worse with higher doses and serum levels of lithium.

Aggravating factors: Use of other medications that also cause tremor, use of caffeine

Progression: It tends to not progress unless, of course, the lithium level changes

Lithium-induced benign tremor: Evaluation

Differentiation from tremor due to lithium toxicity

Lithium toxicity also leads to a tremor. How is that tremor different from lithium-induced benign tremors (Baek et al., 2014)?

1. It has greater amplitude, i.e., is coarser

2. It tends to be more irregular in its rhythm

3. It tends to involve parts of the body other than the hand

4. Other symptoms of lithium toxicity are likely to be present

5. The serum lithium level will usually help. But some patients can have toxicity at lower levels than others.

Ruling out lithium toxicity

1. Examine the patient for location, amplitude, regularity of the tremor

2. Ask and observe for other symptoms of lithium toxicity

3. Order a serum lithium level. In rare cases, an urgent level done on the same day may need to be ordered.

Rule out other causes of tremor

1. In most cases, it is wise to check thyroid function, serum chemistry, and liver function tests.

2. If needed, the mental health clinician may do a brief neurological examination

3. If needed, the patient may be referred to a neurologist for further evaluation.

Documenting the severity of the tremor

If the tremor is determined to be benign, we should document its severity before starting any intervention. This can be done in several ways.

1. Obtaining a sample of handwriting–something standard like the person's name and address, which can be obtained again at follow-up visits.

2. Having the person draw a spiral as discussed above.

Lithium-induced benign tremor: Treatment

Wait-and-watch?

Lithium-induced benign tremor may improve with time without doing anything at all. So, if it has only been present for a few weeks, we may recommend just waiting and watching.

It is important to strongly reassure the patient that even though the tremor is irritating and may be embarrassing, it is not medically harmful. That is, it does not mean that that lithium is harming the body. In my experience, this explanation of the difference between nuisance side effects and medically serious side effects is extremely helpful to patients.

Reduce caffeine

Caffeine definitely makes lithium-induced benign tremor worse. So, the person should be encouraged to gradually wean off caffeine.

Warning! Here is an interesting but potentially confusing situation that may occur. Caffeine also causes diuresis, so when caffeine intake is reduced, the lithium level may increase, which may make the tremor worse rather than better (e.g., Jefferson, 1988)! So, when caffeine is decreased, it should be done gradually, we should monitor the patient clinically, we should consider checking a lithium level, and we should consider lowering the dose of the lithium in order to maintain the same serum level as before.

Reduce the dose of lithium, if possible

Like most side effects, lithium-induced benign tremor is dose related. If reduction in the dose of lithium is clinically feasible, this may reduce the tremor and may even resolve it completely.

However, this is often not a good idea because the prophylactic benefits of lithium are also related to the serum levels. Using too low a dose can mean that the person is being exposed to certain risks without deriving the benefits.

But sometimes it may become unavoidable that some medication be added to treat lithium-induced benign tremor. What are our options and how should we do this?

Note: Anticholinergic medications do NOT work for lithium-induced benign tremor and should not be used for this purpose.

Beta-blockers for lithium-induced benign tremor

Beta blockers are a first-line treatment for essential tremor. And, they have also been shown to be effective for treating lithium-induced benign tremor. This is based on very small controlled clinical trials, multiple published case reports, and many years of clinical experience (Baek et al., 2014).

But which beta blockers may be used to treat lithium-induced benign tremor?

Does the beta blocker need to be centrally-acting?

Now, beta blockers are of two types. Those that are lipophilic and so can enter the brain. These are called "centrally acting." The other type of beta blockers is those that are hydrophilic and do not enter the brain to a significant extent.

For example, propranolol is highly lipophilic, metoprolol is moderately lipophilic, while atenolol is hydrophilic.

Important: In contrast to akathisia, the benefit of beta-blockers for lithium-induced benign tremor is peripheral, not central. Both types of beta-blockers will help.

Nonselective or beta 1 selective beta-blockers?

In this regard, we should know that beta-receptors are of two types: beta 1 and beta 2. On the heart, the beta-receptors are beta 1. On the bronchi, they are beta 2. Some beta-blockers have been developed that are selective for beta 1 receptors. These are sometimes called "cardioselective". But, they will still work for lithium-induced benign tremor.

So, if a person has bronchial asthma but needs a beta-blocker for the treatment of lithium-induced benign tremor, a beta 1 selective medication like metoprolol (Zubenko et al., 1984) or atenolol (Dave, 1989) should be preferred.

Propranolol

Propranolol has been most commonly used for the treatment of lithium-induced benign tremor. However, it should be noted that none of the following characteristics of propranolol are valid reasons for using it in preference to other beta-blockers:

Cost–Many beta-blockers are now generic and cheap

Being centrally-acting–Not needed for treatment of lithium-induced benign tremor

Being non-selective for beta 1 and beta 2 receptors–Also not essential for the treatment of lithium-induced benign tremor.

A typical starting dose is 10 mg three times a day. The dose may be increased, if tolerated, to 20 mg three times a day.

The total daily dose of propranolol for the treatment of tremor is usually 60 to 120 mg/day. Doses up to 360 mg/day may be needed in difficult cases.

Metoprolol

Typical dose: 100 to 200 mg/day

At lower doses, metoprolol is relatively selective for beta-1 receptors but becomes non-selective at higher doses. One small case series found it to be less effective than propranolol when used at lower doses.

Nadolol

Typical dose: 40 to 80 mg/day

Nadolol is infrequently used but may be preferred in cases of significant liver disease (e.g., Dave and Langbart, 1994).

Antiepileptic medications for lithium-induced benign tremor?

Unfortunately, lithium-induced benign tremor has hardly been studied. All we have to go on is:

1. Case reports/case series of a medication to treat lithium-induced benign tremor

2. Medications that are known to be effective in essential tremor and so may work for lithium-induced benign tremor.

The table below shows which antiepileptics have been reported to be effective for the treatment of essential tremor, lithium-induced benign tremor, or both. Due to lack of a proven options, even case reports are mentioned in this table.

Medication	Effectiveness for Essential Tremor	Effectiveness for Lithium-Induced Benign Tremor
Primidone	First-line	Case report (Goumentouk et al., 1989)
Pregabalin	Second-line	Case report (Marks et al., 2008)
Topiramate	Second-line	None
Gabapentin	Second-line	None

Vitamin B6 (pyridoxine) for lithium-induced benign tremor?

Note: I use the term "lithium-induced benign tremor" to distinguish this from the tremor that may occur due to lithium toxicity.

Unfortunately, lithium-induced benign tremor has hardly been studied. All we have to go on is:

1. Case reports/case series/open-label trials of a medication to treat lithium-induced benign tremor

2. Medications that are known to be effective in essential tremor and so may work for lithium-induced benign tremor.

Might vitamin B6 (pyridoxine) work?

A small open-label clinical trial (only five patients; Miodownik et al., 2002) and a case series (seven patients; Dias Alves et al., 2017) have been published of the use of vitamin B6 for the treatment of lithium-induced benign tremors.

In the small open-label clinical trial, four out of five patients showed substantial improvement after being treated for four weeks with vitamin B6 (Miodownik et al., 2002).

In the other case series, seven patients with lithium-induced benign tremor were treated with vitamin B6 (pyridoxine) of whom two had complete resolution and another three had partial improvement in the tremor (Dias Alves et al., 2017).

Note: It has not been shown in a randomized, double-blind, controlled clinical trial that vitamin B6 (pyridoxine) is effective for lithium-induced benign tremor.

What might the mechanism of action be?

Vitamin B6 was tried for lithium-induced benign tremor because it had been tried for parkinsonism and tardive dyskinesia. But, its mechanism of action is not known. It is speculated that it may be due to its antioxidant effects (Dias Alves et al., 2017).

How much?

750 to 1200 mg/day of pyridoxine

How long should the trial be?

The open-label clinical trial was predetermined to last four weeks. But, the duration of treatment was flexible in the case series (Dias Alves et al., 2017). In those patients, it took between 6 to 150 days before the benefit was seen.

These observations suggest that while pyridoxine may work in four weeks or so, if it is tried off-label for this purpose, it may need to be tried for a few months before concluding that it did not work.

For how long should the pyridoxine be continued if it does work?

In one case series, the tremors came back in three of four patients after the vitamin B6 was stopped (Miodownik et al., 2002). In the other case series, in all cases, when the pyridoxine was stopped in patients in whom it had worked, the tremor came back (Dias Alves et al., 2017).

These observations suggest that the vitamin B6 may need to be continued for a long time. BUT, as discussed below, long-term treatment with high dose vitamin B6 may lead to toxicity. So, the patient should be carefully monitored clinically and with measurement of plasma levels of vitamin B6.

Potential side effects?

In the open-label study and case series discussed above, no side effects attributable to vitamin B6 were reported (Miodownik et al., 2002; Dias Alves et al., 2017).

But, it is not true that B vitamins cannot be toxic because they are water soluble and will just get excreted. In high doses (similar to or higher than those recommended for lithium-induced benign tremor) given for a long time, pyridoxine can be toxic. The adverse effects that have been reported included:

— Nausea

— Dizziness

— Acne

— Tingling in the skin

— Photosensitivity and rash in areas exposed to the sun

— Sensory neuropathy (e.g., Schaumburg et al., 1983)

— Sensorimotor neuropathy (e.g., Kulkantrakorn, 2014)

— At extremely high doses, pyridoxine can also cause motor neuropathy (e.g., Morra et al., 1993).

References: See https://simpleandpractical.com/side-effects-references

CHAPTER 15: SKIN

ACNE

Use of lithium has been associated with many different kinds of skin problems. Among these is an increased risk of both new onset of acne AND worsening of pre-existing acne.

To be more exact, drug-induced acne can be called an "acneiform eruption", meaning that it is "acne-like" or similar in some ways to acne vulgaris.

Note: When we commonly talk of "acne", we mean "acne vulgaris". That's the acne you may have had when you were a teenager. Remember that?

Acne vulgaris is different from acne rosacea (also just called "rosacea").

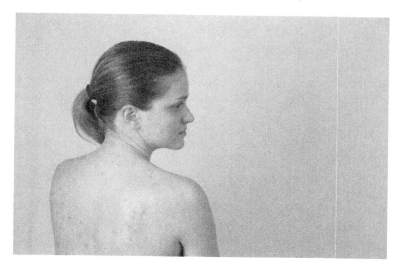

Why is this important?

Acne is socially embarrassing to patients. In my clinical experience, side effects that are socially embarrassing are more likely to lead to the patient stopping the medication.

Lithium-related acne is known to be an important cause of stopping lithium especially in young adults (Yeung and Chan, 2004).

How common is it?

This is not clearly known. Very different prevalence rates (from 3% to 45%) have been reported (Yeung and Chan, 2004).

Who is at greater risk?

1. Males

2. Higher doses of lithium. This is relevant because it means that lowering the dose of the lithium, if possible, may reduce the severity of the acne.

3. Past history of severe acne

4. Family history of severe acne

Clinical features

If a person has acne, how do we know that it may be due to the lithium?

1. Timing: The acne typically begins a few weeks after first starting the lithium (Yeung and Chan, 2004) and usually within the first six months.

2. Parts of the body: Lithium-related acne tends to be more prominent on the limbs and trunk rather than on the face (Yeung and Chan, 2004).

Also, while variations are possible, lithium-induced acne tends to be:

3. Monomorphic, i.e., all the lesions are similar. Acne vulgaris that is not caused by medications tends to be polymorphic, i.e., with many different types of lesions.

4. Papular or pustular. A papule is a "bump" that is small (less than 0.5 cm). A pustule is a similar raised lesion except that it has pus in it.

5. Lacking in comedones ("blackheads") or cysts

6. Persistent and non-cyclical. That is, the lesions tend to stay the same rather than go through a clear evolution and changes which is typical for spontaneous acne.

Management of lithium-related acne

1. Lithium-related acne is probably dose-related, so lowering the dose (if possible) should be considered.

2. The treatments for acne that work when it is not due to lithium seem to work for lithium-related acne as well.

Warning! Tetracycline is a commonly used antibiotic for the treatment of acne. But, it should be avoided in persons on lithium because it interacts with lithium.

Warning! Isotretinoin for acne has been associated with a risk of destabilization of the bipolar disorder (Schaffer et al., 2010).

3. But sometimes there may be no alternative except to stop lithium. In such cases, we must remember to taper the lithium gradually rather than stopping it rather abruptly.

The acne tends to improve about a month after the lithium dose is reduced or the lithium is stopped (Yeung and Chan, 2004), but it can take a few months to resolve (e.g., Scarfi and Arunachalam, 2013).

EXCESSIVE SWEATING (HYPERHIDROSIS)

Antidepressant-induced excessive sweating (ADIES) or Hyperhidrosis

Excessive sweating or hyperhidrosis can be associated with several psychiatric and non-psychiatric medications. Antidepressant-induced excessive sweating (ADIES) can occur with all or almost all antidepressants including tricyclic antidepressants, selective serotonin reuptake inhibitors (SSRIs), serotonin-norepinephrine reuptake inhibitors (SNRIs), and bupropion.

Really? Is this is a common problem?

Everyone asks me: is this a common problem? Well, we can look at a few different sources to estimate how often ADIES occurs.

The rates for ADIES with different antidepressants reported in the Physician's Desk Reference (www.pdr.net) vary from 5% to 14% of patients on an SSRI or SNRI, which is at least twice as often as on placebo.

A meta-analysis of clinical trials of SSRIs found that about 10% of patients reported sweating as an adverse event.

Combining these two sources above, we can say that excessive sweating occurs in about 10% of patients on antidepressants.

A study in routine clinical settings but using systematic assessment for adverse events associated with a variety of antidepressants found exces-sive sweating in 8.3% (moclobemide) to 40% (bupropion) of patients.

Why ADIES is important

Besides being common, ADIES causes significant distress to patients and can cause functional impairment as well. Patients often have to make changes to their activities and lifestyle because of the excessive sweating.

ADIES can be bothersome to patients in a variety of ways: the clothes feeling and appearing wet, visible sweat that needs to be wiped off repeatedly, sweating so badly that droplets of sweat drop off the body. The sweating can make patients very uncomfortable, make patients irritable, and interfere with their sleep. In addition, it can be embarrassing, lead to patients avoiding going out, and cause patients to change their clothes repeatedly.

While there is little data on this, ADIES can lead to non-adherence with antidepressants in some patients. Treating ADIES, if treatment is needed, can have a positive effect on patients' well being.

Antidepressant-induced excessive sweating (ADIES) or Hyperhidrosis: Clinical features

In the previous section, we noted that antidepressant-induced excessive sweating is a relatively common side effect but is often not recognized or treated.

Problem: often, patients don't realize that the excessive sweating is due to the antidepressants. Worse problem: when patients report the excessive sweating to clinicians, due to clinicians' lack of familiarity with this adverse effect, they are often told that it is not due to the antidepressant.C

Our published study on ADIES (Mago et al., 2013) was the first study to describe the clinical features of ADIES. Excessive sweating associated with antidepressants appears to have a clinical presentation that differs in some ways from sweating due to warm temperatures and to anxiety. Rather than the armpits and palms, ADIES tends to be particularly was prominent in the upper body, face, scalp, neck, and chest. ADIES tends to occur in bursts that may also be superimposed on a baseline increase in sweating. Nearly half of patients who present with ADIES report that indicated that they tended to sweat more than other people even before they started taking an antidepressant. About a third of patients with ADIES report a family history of excessive sweating, either with or without the family member being on an antidepressant.

ADIES can be bothersome to patients in a variety of ways: the clothes feeling and appearing wet, visible sweat that needs to be wiped off repeatedly, sweating so badly that droplets of sweat drop off the body. The sweating can make patients very uncomfortable, make patients irritable, and interfere with their sleep. In addition, it can be embarrassing, lead to patients avoiding going out, and cause patients to change their clothes repeatedly.

Antidepressant-induced excessive sweating (ADIES) or Hyperhidrosis: Management

While wait-and-watch may be reasonable in the first few weeks or months, in large numbers of patients, ADIES persists for as long as the antidepressant is taken.

Use of antiperspirants is of little help to patients with ADIES since much of the sweating occurs on the scalp, face, and upper chest — areas of the body where it antiperspirants are not usually applied.

ADIES is dose-related, so if a reduction in dose of the antidepressant is clinically feasible, it should be tried. This may or may not reduce or remove the problem.

As noted above, some antidepressants are more likely to cause ADIES than others. If this is feasible, changing from bupropion or an SNRI to an SSRI (other than paroxetine) may solve the problem in some cases.

Even among the SSRIs, it is possible that ADIES (like other adverse effects) may occur with one SSRI but not another. So, while the ADIES often occurs with the other SSRI as well, if clinically appropriate, a trial of changing to another SSRI is an option.

We often encounter situations where a particular antidepressant (e.g., an SNRI) has been very helpful while other antidepressants have not, but the patient has ADIES on this antidepressant. This situation also occurs where bupropion is the culprit but the patient wants to continue on bupropion because it is the only one that has not caused significant sexual dysfunction. In such difficult situations, it becomes necessary and appropriate to add another medication (an "antidote") to treat the ADIES.

Usually, in the sympathetic nervous system the neurotransmitter is norepinephrine and in the parasympathetic nervous system, it is acetylcholine. However, the sweat glands are unique in that in their innervation, the upper neurons that end at sympathetic ganglia utilize norepinephrine as the neurotransmitter while the lower neurons that end on the sweat glands release acetylcholine. The reason for reminding you of these facts is that we can treat ADIES by either blocking the effect of norepinephrine on post-synaptic alpha-1 receptors or by blocking the effect of acetylcholine on post-synaptic muscarinic receptors.

Case reports have suggested the potential use of several different medications for the treatment of ADIES. Terazosin, an alpha-1 blocker, is the only medication that has been shown in clinical trials (the first one being our study published in 2013) to be effective for ADIES. In our uncontrolled study, 22 of 23 patients were "much improved" or "very much improved" on terazosin. Terazosin was prescribed in a dose of 1 mg at bedtime and increased at weekly intervals to 4 to 6 mg at bedtime. The commonest adverse effects of terazosin were dizziness/lightheadedness (9 of 23 patients) and dry mouth (4 of 23 patients). Importantly, terazosin is associated with a risk of hypotension, especially orthostatic. Serious hypotension with the first dose has been reported to occasionally occur as well, though this did not occur in any patient in our study. Clonidine is another anti-adrenergic medication that has been shown to be effective in case reports. Another potential approach to treating ADIES is to use an anticholinergic. Anticholinergics do appear to work in published case reports. However, one barrier to using anticholinergics like benztropine to treat ADIES is that they can cause significant cognitive impairment. One patient to whom I prescribed benztropine to treat ADIES reported feeling significantly "clouded" and impaired at his work. In an attempt to avoid this problem, glycopyrrolate (Robinul®) is sometimes used because it does not cross the blood-brain barrier to a significant extent. In 2013, I published the first case of the use of glycopyrrolate to treat ADIES but it has not been studied in a clinical trial (as of May 2018).

Glycopyrrolate should be started at 1 mg twice and day and increased to a usual maximum of 6 mg/day in three divided doses. Its benefits last for only a few hours. The timing of the medication can be adjusted according to the time of the day when the greatest ADIES is expected. If the excessive sweating is intermittent, e.g., when the patient only experiences it when intermittently not in air conditioning, glycopyrrolate can also be used as needed (prn).

We have to counsel patients that terazosin or glycopyrrolate do not "cure" the excessive sweating, but provide symptom relief. We should also tell them that if the terazosin or glycopyrrolate is stopped, the benefits do not disappear right away. Therefore, this does not mean that they don't need the medication. The excessive sweating may take a few days or even months to come back. On the other hand, the excessive sweating tends to vary depending on the ambient temperature. Therefore, in the winter or if patients will mainly stay indoors with air-conditioning, the dose of the medication can be reduced. It is very important with terazosin not to stop or start the medication suddenly since serious hypotension or rebound hypertension can occur.

HAIR LOSS (ALOPECIA)

Valproate and hair loss (alopecia)

1. It is not rare.

Hair loss or alopecia can occur in a significant percentage of people taking valproate. The estimated percentage is somewhere between 4% and 12% (McKinney et al., 1996; Chen et al., 2015), or even more.

2. It is dose-dependent

Hair loss associated with valproate is often reported in those with a higher serum level, e.g., 100 mcg/mL (Tomita et al., 2015; Ramakrishnappa and Belhekar, 2013). That the prevalence of alopecia increases with dose is also supported by studies in rats (Korkmazer et al., 2006).

The importance of knowing this is that dose reduction may help if valproate-induced hair loss occurs (e.g., Fatemi and Calabrese, 1995).

3. It is diffuse and non-scarring

Like other drug-induced hair loss, that occurring with valproate is also diffuse rather than patchy and it is not associated with scarring (Ramakrishnappa and Belhekar, 2013).

4. It is usually reversible, but…

After stopping valproate, the hair usually grows back.

However, the new hair may be curly! Some like this and some don't.

In rare cases, the new hair may be of a different color (Herranz et al., 1981).

5. It may be caused by interference with mineral absorption

Valproate treatment may decrease levels of zinc, selenium, copper, etc (Hurd et al., 1984). However, routinely checking levels is not recommended because zinc levels, while lower than at baseline, are generally still within normal range (Castro-Gago et al., 2011).

6. Its risk may be affected by what time valproate is taken

Valproate should be not be given close to the time when supplements like vitamins, zinc, folate, and biotin are taken; this may reduce the risk of hair loss.

7. Lastly, here are some potential treatments…

Zinc 15 mg/day and selenium 150 mcg/day were reported to reverse hair loss in one patient (Fatemi and Calabrese, 1995). I have also used the combination of zinc and selenium with success. Others have recommended different doses, e.g., 25 to 50 mg/day of zinc and 20 mcg/day of selenium.

Supplementation of biotin 10 mg/day should also be considered (Korkmazer et al., 2006; Grootens et al., 2017).

SKIN REACTIONS

How common are benign and serious rashes with lamotrigine?

Patients rightfully want to know and should be told the chances of having a serious allergic reaction that is accompanied by a skin rash, i.e., Stevens-Johnson syndrome (SJS) or toxic epidermal necrolysis (TEN). What do you tell your patients? What is the percentage chance of a "serious rash"?

But, while patients must take any new onset of rash very seriously, in order that they don't completely freak out when they get a skin rash, they should also be told that getting a different kind of rash–a "benign rash"–is much more common than getting a "serious rash".

The Prescribing Information for brand name Lamictal carries a boxed warning ("black box warning") that includes the statement:

"LAMICTAL® can cause serious rashes requiring hospitalization and discontinuation of treatment. The incidence of these rashes, which have included Stevens-Johnson syndrome, is approximately 0.3% to 0.8% in pediatric patients (aged 2 to 17 years) and 0.08% to 0.3% in adults receiving LAMICTAL." (emphasis added).

The higher end of that range, 0.3%, would mean that up to 1 in every 330 patients gets a serious rash. That is not what has been found in the widespread clinical use of lamotrigine. But these numbers included patients who were treated for epilepsy.

What about in clinical trials of patients treated with lamotrigine for bipolar disorder? In a systematic review of all randomized controlled trials published in English (Bloom and Amber, 2017), nearly 10,000 patients with bipolar disorder received lamotrigine. The incidence of skin reactions was about 9% while the incidence of SJS/TEN was 0.02%.

So, while it is hard to give the patient an exact number as to the risk of a serious rash, what I say is:

"It is not clear what are the exact chances of a person getting a serious rash, but it is about 1 in 1000. It is possible that it may be lower than that, like 1 in 5000"

Then I continue by saying, "It is much, much more likely that you could get a benign skin rash than a serious rash. Your chances of getting a benign skin reaction are about 1 in 10."

Dermatological precautions when starting lamotrigine

Could certain precautions related to not doing anything that might irritate the skin lead to a lower incidence of non-serious skin rash with lamotrigine?

The benefit of such dermatological precautions is unproven. The one controlled study that looked at this question (Ketter et al., 2006), did not find any reduction in the incidence of benign rash.

But, these precautions are harmless and relatively easy to implement. I still tell my patients that we want to try to minimize the risk of rash due to any reason other than the medication (e.g., allergic reaction to a new skin product, sunburn) that may cause confusion and unnecessarily lead to the lamotrigine being permanently stopped.

What precautions?

1. Lamotrigine should not be started within two weeks of having a rash, viral illness, or vaccination.

2. For the first three months after starting lamotrigine, the patient should avoid using any new medicine or food.

3. For the first three months after starting lamotrigine, the patient should

avoid using any new product that comes in contact with the skin and could cause a rash, e.g., cosmetic, deodorant, detergent, fabric softener, etc. Products that the patient has been using for a while can, of course, be continued.

4. For the first three months after starting lamotrigine, the patient should also avoid getting sunburn or exposure to poison ivy.

Restarting lamotrigine: A case study

All patients should be given the instruction that if they stop lamotrigine for more than three to five days or more for any reason, they must not restart it at their usual dose. They must call us and need to be started again using the initial dosing schedule, which is usually 25 mg/day for 2 weeks and so on.

To emphasize how important this instruction is, here is a published case (Jangir et al., 2011) in which restarting lamotrigine at the original dose after an interruption of a few months led disaster.

The patient was a woman with bipolar disorder, depressed who reached remission on lamotrigine 200 mg/day and escitalopram 20 mg/day. She then discontinued medication on her own; unfortunately, many of our patients do that.

After four months, depressive symptoms recurred, so she started taking the same medications on her own, without consulting with her doctor. She started directly on the lamotrigine 200 mg/day she was taking in the previous episode. Is it possible that this could happen with one of our own patients? Of course, it is possible.

Within 7 to 10 days, she developed skin eruptions that progressed to Stevens-Johnson syndrome. Here are the photos from that case:

.

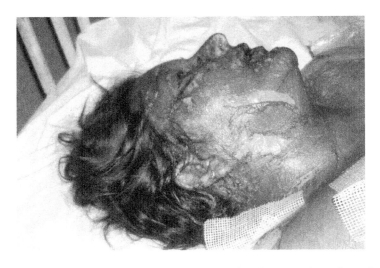

Figure 1: Large areas of epidermal shedding, and red and exquisitely tender underlying denuded skin over the trunk, neck, face, ear and extremities

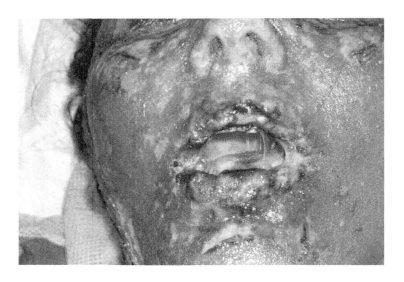

Figure 2: Massive erosions and aphthous ulcers on oral mucosa and tongue and hemorrhagic crusting over the lips.

The moral of the story is that we must tell all patients who are started on lamotrigine that if they stop or miss the lamotrigine for more than three to five days, they must NOT restart it at the original dose. They should call us for instructions and we should start the titration again from 25 mg/day. This may be frustrating to the patient and to us, but it needs to be done.

Dermatological precautions when starting lamotrigine

Could certain precautions related to not doing anything that might irritate the skin lead to a lower incidence of non-serious skin rash with lamotrigine?

The benefit of such dermatological precautions is unproven. The one controlled study that looked at this question (Ketter et al., 2006), did not find any reduction in the incidence of benign rash.

But, these precautions are harmless and relatively easy to implement. I still tell my patients that we want to try to minimize the risk of rash due to any reason other than the medication (e.g., allergic reaction to a new skin product, sunburn) that may cause confusion and unnecessarily lead to the lamotrigine being permanently stopped.

What precautions?

1. Lamotrigine should not be started within two weeks of having a rash, viral illness, or vaccination.

2. For the first three months after starting lamotrigine, the patient should avoid using any new medicine or food.

3.For the first three months after starting lamotrigine, the patient should avoid using any new product that comes in contact with the skin and could cause a rash, e.g., cosmetic, deodorant, detergent, fabric softener, etc. Products that the patient has been using for a while can, of course, be continued.

3. For the first three months after starting lamotrigine, the patient should also avoid getting sunburn or exposure to poison ivy.

Benign or dangerous skin rash?

It is a relatively common clinical problem that we need to decide whether a skin rash in a person taking lamotrigine is likely to be benign or serious, i.e., indicating onset of Steven-Johnson Syndrome (SJS) or Toxic Epidermal Necrolysis (TEN).

Note: The clinical features noted below are not a guarantee that the rash is benign. They are provided here for general educational purposes and are only one part of the assessment by a medical professional, not a substitute for medical assessment. Due to the seriousness of SJS/ TEN, it is recommended that we err on the side of caution.

Why is this a common problem?

A benign rash occurs in about 6% of people on lamotrigine while SJS occurs in 0.1% or less of people. So, we are much, much more likely to see a benign rash than SJS.

It is easy for textbooks to say: "Consultation with a dermatologist is recommended", but not so easy to get a person to see a dermatologist within 24 hours.

Features suggestive of serious rash (SJS/ TEN)

If any of the following are present, it makes Stevens-Johnson Syndrome (SJS) /Toxic Epidermal Necrolysis (TEN) more likely. These features can be asked of the person and/or specifically looked for during examination of the person.

1. Systemic symptoms

Typically, the fever and flu-like symptoms occur first, then a rash appears which progresses rapidly. The systemic symptoms may include fever, malaise, anorexia, headache, rhinitis, sore throat, cough, pain the muscles of the joints, etc. We should remember that the rash of Stevens-Johnson Syndrome is really part of a systemic hypersensitivity reaction.

2. Mucosal involvement

There is pain or a lesion in the nose, mouth, eyes, while urinating or defecating, or in the penis or vagina. That is, any symptoms or signs of involvement of a mucosal surface or conjunctiva. The mucosal involvement often begins with painful, burning sensations of the lips, conjunctivae, and genitalia (Dodiuk-Gad et al., 2015).

3. Facial involvement

The rash involves the face or the face is swollen.

4. Characteristics of the rash

The rash is typically dark red in color, irregularly shaped, expands, becomes confluent (the different areas of rash are coming together), and spreads to the other areas. The rash may include red or purple spots in the skin or mucous membranes (purpura).

5. Peeling off

There are blisters or the skin is peeling off in any area of the rash, including on the palms and soles. If spontaneous detachment of the epidermis is not seen, put lateral pressure with a finger on a red area of the rash. If the epidermis separates, this is called a positive Nikolsky sign. A red, sometimes oozing dermis may be exposed (Dodiuk-Gad et al., 2015).

6. Pain

The rash is painful to touch.

7. Lymph glands

On examination, the lymph glands in the neck, axilla, and groin are enlarged.

8. Laboratory tests

If the symptoms and signs suggest the possibility of SJS/ TEN, laboratory tests can help in assessing the person. The WBC count and hepatic enzymes (AST and ALT) may be elevated. There may be microscopic hematuria.

Next steps

1. If the patient is not in your office, ask the person to take photos of the rash and send them to you.

2. In case of doubt, consider asking the person to immediately go to the emergency room.

Non-drug causes of Stevens-Johnson Syndrome (SJS)/Toxic Epidermal Necrolysis (TEN)

The great majority of cases of Stevens-Johnson Syndrome (SJS) or Toxic Epidermal Necrolysis (TEN) are due to a hypersensitivity reaction to a medication (Schwartz et al., 2013).

Some of the rest are idiopathic and some are believed to be associated with non-drug causes.

Infectious causes of SJS/ TEN

Some of the rare, infectious causes of SJS/ TEN are listed below. But, infections may be more likely to be associated with SJS/ TEN in children than in adults (Léauté-Labrèze et al., 2000). Of these, infection with Mycoplasma pneumoniae may be the most common infectious cause (Mulvey et al., 2007).

– Cytomegalovirus (e.g., Cruz et al., 2010; Khalaf et al., 2011)

– Dengue virus (e.g., Grieb et al., 2010)

– Herpes simplex (e.g., Detjen et al., 1992; Golden et al., 1993; Aihara et al., 2004)

– Measles-Mumps-Rubella or other vaccinations (Ball et al., 2001)

– Mycoplasma pneumonia (e.g., Fournier et al., 1995; Mulvey et al., 2007)

– Varicella (e.g., Bay et al., 2005)

Note: It is much more likely that infections like herpes or varicella are associated with erythema multiforme, which is a benign, self-limiting condition. It is important to be able to differentiate between erythema multiforme and SJS/ TEN.

Other causes of SJS/ TEN

– Contrast medium, like that used during coronary angiography (e.g., Garza et al., 2005; Baldwin et al., 2010)

Do past infections increase the risk of Stevens-Johnson Syndrome (SJS) / Toxic Epidermal Necrolysis (TEN)?

Question: Is there an increased risk of Stevens-Johnson Syndrome in patients with a history of herpes or other viral infections?

This is a difficult question but we do have a tentative answer. The reason this question is important is that mental health clinicians want to know if they should either avoid psychotropic medications (e.g., lamotrigine, carbamazepine, modafinil) that have been associated with Stevens-Johnson Syndrome (SJS) or Toxic Epidermal Necrolysis (TEN) in patients with certain infections (current or past) or discuss the increased risk with the patient.

Reactivation of a past infection

In rare cases, Stevens-Johnson syndrome has been reported to occur with reactivation of herpes simplex infection. For example, a case was reported in which Stevens-Johnson syndrome recurred and became progressively more severe over several years, being precipitated each time with herpes simplex virus infection of the mouth (Detjen et al., 1992). This patient was successfully managed by a strategy including early treatment of the herpes recurrences with acyclovir (Cheriyan and Patterson, 1996).

SJS/ TEN has also been associated with reactivation of prior cytomegalovirus infection (Tagajdid et al., 2013).

So, in answer to the above question–yes, there is some risk of SJS/ TEN with various infections and, rarely, this could be associated with infections that tend to recur or be reactivated (e.g., herpes, cytomegalovirus).

Both reactivation of infection AND starting a new medication

To make things more complicated, in some reported cases, SJS/ TEN was associated with starting a drug AND reactivation of an infection (Tagajdid et al., 2013).

So, in patients with a history of herpes or cytomegalovirus, there may a slightly greater risk of SJS/ TEN when a medication that has been associated with SJS/ TEN is started, compared with starting on a medication with no such history of infection. To what extent the risk is increased is not possible to say.

References: See https://simpleandpractical.com/side-effects-references

CHAPTER 16: SLEEP

INSOMNIA

MAO inhibitor-induced insomnia

MAO inhibitors can lead to a feeling of being overstimulated during the day and to insomnia at night. While daytime hyperstimulation may be more likely to occur with tranylcypromine, insomnia occurs with both phenelzine and tranylcypromine (Remick et al., 1989).

What can we do?

1. Recommend taking more of the medication earlier in the day rather than close to bedtime.

2. Consider dose reduction, if possible

3. If hyperstimulation during the day is also present in addition to the insomnia AND the person is on tranylcypromine, consider switching to phenelzine.

Warning! Switching from one MAO inhibitor to another requires a washout period. See Switching from one MAO inhibitor to another.

4. A standard hypnotic may be used (e.g., zolpidem)

5. A low dose of trazodone (i..e, about 50 to 100 mg at bedtime) can be used. There is published data supporting the safe use of an MAO inhibitor along with a low dose of trazodone (e.g., Nierenberg and Keck, 1989; Jacobsen, 1990)

6. A low dose of a sedating tricyclic antidepressant (e.g., trimipramine, amitriptyline) can be used, but clomipramine, a particularly serotonergic drug, should not be be combined with an MAO inhibitor.

Warning! Trazodone and tricyclic antidepressants are listed as being contraindicated with MAO inhibitors.

However, there is published data and clinical experience supporting the use of an MAO inhibitor along with trazodone or a tricyclic antidepressant (other than clomipramine), which is summarized HERE.

7. Low dose quetiapine (i.e., about 50 mg at bedtime) has also been used to treat insomnia due to an MAO inhibitor (case report only: Sokolski and Brown, 2006).

References

Jacobsen FM. Low-dose trazodone as a hypnotic in patients treated with MAOIs and other psychotropics: a pilot study. J Clin Psychiatry. 1990 Jul;51(7):298-302. PubMed PMID: 2365668.

Nierenberg AA, Keck PE Jr. Management of monoamine oxidase inhibitor-associated insomnia with trazodone. J Clin Psychopharmacol. 1989 Feb;9(1):42-5. PubMed PMID: 2708555.

Remick RA, Froese C, Keller FD. Common side effects associated with monoamine oxidase inhibitors. Prog Neuropsychopharmacol Biol Psychiatry. 1989;13(3-4):497-504. PubMed PMID: 2748873.

Sokolski KN, Brown BJ. Quetiapine for insomnia associated with refractory depression exacerbated by phenelzine. Ann Pharmacother. 2006 Mar;40(3):567-70. Epub 2006 Feb 14. PubMed PMID: 16478812.

CHAPTER 17: URINARY SYSTEM

KIDNEY STONES

Warning! Topiramate can cause kidney stones

Some mental health clinicians frequently prescribe topiramate, mainly due to its propensity to cause weight loss. I am not one of them. For many reasons, I rarely prescribe topiramate. One of the reasons is that it can cause kidney stones—typically, calcium phosphate and calcium oxalate (Jion et al., 2015).

But, don't most medicines have a potential risk of some serious side effect or another? We still prescribe them, don't we? Yes, but we also have to keep in mind how often that serious side effect can occur.

How often do kidney stones occur with topiramate?

A psychopharmacology expert once asked me if I may be overemphasizing the risk of stone formation with topiramate, which, he said, is quite rare. So, let's look at data on how often urinary system stones occur in patients on topiramate.

The *Prescribing Information* for topiramate (brand name Topamax®) notes:

" During adjunctive epilepsy trials, the risk for kidney stones in [topiramate]-treated adults was 1.5%, an incidence about 2 to 4 times greater than expected in a similar, untreated population."

In my opinion, for a serious side effect like kidney stones, 1.5% is a fairly high number. Do you agree?

If you pause to think about it, you will realize that since most kidney stones are asymptomatic, if we did ultrasounds on patients, we would find many more people with kidney stones.

Laboratory findings related to stone formation in patients on topiramate

Topiramate is an inhibitor of carbonic anhydrase, an enzyme involved in acid-base regulation. Inhibition of carbonic anhydrase leads to increased excretion of bicarbonate in the urine. This makes the urine more alkaline (increased pH) and the blood more acidic (metabolic acidosis).

These effects, in turn, lead to some key changes in the urine that promote stone formation:

1. Hypercalciuria, which is a fancy way of saying "increased calcium in the urine". More calcium in the urine, obviously, increases the risk of the formation of calcium-containing stones.

2. Hypocitraturia, which is a fancy way of saying "decreased citrate in the urine". It is well-documented that topiramate is consistently associated with hypocitraturia.

What has citrate got to do with stone formation? Citrate forms a soluble complex with calcium and so it tends to prevent stone formation even when urinary calcium is high (Jion et al., 2015). That's why hypocitraturia is associated with a higher incidence of both calcium phosphate stones and calcium oxalate stones (Corbin Bush et al., 2013). Potassium citrate is used as a treatment to prevent the recurrence of calcium-containing stones.

Though this is not a routine part of monitoring in patients on topiramate, if needed, the patient's urine can be tested for pH, calcium/creatinine ratio, and citrate/creatinine ratio (Corbin Bush et al., 2013). By evaluating calcium and citrate in the urine as a ratio against creatinine, we can use a single urine sample rather than a 24-hour urine sample, which is a pain in the behind to collect.

In one study in children taking topiramate (Corbin Bush et al.., 2013):

– About 70% had a pH of > 6.7

– About 50% had hypercalciuria, and

– About 95% had hypocitraturia.

What factors may increase the risk further?

1. Males

The Prescribing Information notes: "As in the general population, the incidence of stone formation among [topiramate]-treated patients was higher in men."

2. History of urinary stones

Before prescribing topiramate, we should ask about any history of urinary stones in the past. But, even if there is a history of urinary stones in the patient, this is not an absolute contraindication to using topiramate. It depends on:

– Whether we know what factors may have led that person to develop urinary stones

– Whether or not those factors are still present.

3. Dose

In clinical trials of topiramate, the incidence of kidney stones was 0% with placebo, 0% with 50 mg/day, 1% with 100 mg/day, and 2% with 200 mg/day (Marmura, 2014).

4. Using topiramate along with another medication that is also a carbonic anhydrase inhibitor, e.g., zonisamide, acetazolamide.

The Prescribing Information for topiramate notes that the use of topiramate should be avoided in persons on other carbonic anhydrase inhibitors.

5. Ketogenic diet

The Prescribing Information for topiramate notes that the use of topiramate should be avoided in persons on a ketogenic diet.

6. Low fluid intake

Since increased urinary volume decreases the concentration of substances involved in stone formation, adequate hydration may reduce stone formation (Prescribing Information). So, for all patients who are being started on topiramate (or who are already on topiramate), we should tell them to make sure they drink an adequate amount of fluids every day.

How can patients know if they are drinking an adequate amount of fluids? Here are two simple tips:

− If the patient's urine is either colorless like water or very pale yellow, the patient's fluid intake is pretty good.

− I typically tell my patients that whenever they pee and the urine is not colorless or very pale yellow, they should drink a cup of water when they come out of the bathroom.

POLYURIA AND DIABETES INSIPIDUS

Lithium-induced polyuria and diabetes insipidus

Polyuria is excessive production of urine—more than 2.5 L/day and even up to 8 L/day. Polyuria may progress to diabetes insipidus. Both polyuria and diabetes insipidus are among the most common side effects of lithium. Polyuria occurs in up to 70% of patients on lithium and diabetes insipidus occurs in between 10 to 20% of patients.

Why are they important?

These conditions are troublesome to the patient, may affect medication adherence, and in rare cases may lead to irreversible tubular dysfunction.

However, active efforts to screen for and manage polyuria/diabetes insipidus are not commonly undertaken.

How lithium causes diabetes insipidus

Normally, antidiuretic hormone (ADH; also known as vasopressin) acts on the distal and collecting tubules of the kidney to reabsorb most of the water that was filtered out into the urine. By increasing or decreasing this reabsorption, the body controls the amount of urine produced.

But, this process may be impaired due to two main reasons: impaired production of ADH by the pituitary (called central diabetes insipidus) or impairment in the kidney's responsiveness to ADH (called nephrogenic diabetes insipidus).

Lithium impairs the effect of antidiuretic hormone on the distal and collecting tubules. This leads to excessively dilute urine. So, what lithium can cause is nephrogenic diabetes insipidus.

Lithium-induced polyuria and diabetes insipidus: Evaluation

Urine volume

We should ask all patients on long-term lithium treatment whether they are urinating more than they used to and how often they have to wake up at night to urinate. We should remember that polyuria occurs in 50 to 70% of patients on long-term lithium treatment.

When interviewing the patient about this issue, we should keep in mind that it is the quantity of urine that we are asking about rather than the frequency of urinating.

Waking up at night more than once to urinate may suggest polyuria unless there is another cause like prostate enlargement.

In case of doubt, a 24-hour urine sample can be collected to measure the volume of urine produced over 24 hours (Gitlin, 1999). But how much urine is too much?

Greater than 3 liters in 24 hours is the generally accepted cut off for polyuria (Makaryus and McFarlane, 2006). This is useful to know.

Fluid intake

We should also ask the patient how much fluid he or she is consuming. In case of doubt, we can have the patient measure the amount of fluid being consumed. Let's make sure that the polyuria is not simply due to polydipsia.

Laboratory tests

Urine osmolality and a basic metabolic panel should be ordered to help determine the cause of the polyuria.

1. In polyuria due to diabetes mellitus, the urine osmolality is 300 mOsmol/kg or more and the serum glucose is elevated.

2. But, in polyuria due to diabetes insipidus, the urine osmolality is low, less than 200 mOsmol/kg, even though the person is not drinking excessive amounts of fluid.

Also, in severe cases of diabetes insipidus, the serum sodium may be elevated.

But the diabetes insipidus could be central (due to inadequate production of ADH/vasopressin) or nephrogenic (due to the kidney not responding to the ADH). The only way to differentiate between the two is to refer the patient for a water deprivation/desmopressin test, which we will discuss

Water deprivation/ Desmopressin test

It is rare for mental health patients to need this and lithium must be stopped before water deprivation is attempted. However, in case one of our patients needs to be referred for this, we should know that the gold standard test to differentiate nephrogenic diabetes insipidus from psychogenic polydipsia and central diabetes insipidus (due to lack of ADH/vasopressin secretion) is water deprivation followed by injection of desmopressin.

If this test is needed, it should be done, not by us, but only by a physician experienced in doing it.

In nephrogenic diabetes, even after water deprivation, the urine osmolality remains below plasma osmolality (Makaryus and McFarlane, 2006). That is, the kidney is unable to adequately concentrate the urine even when there is a need to conserve water.

Then, desmopressin (a synthetic analog of ADH/vasopressin) is injected, but there is a limited response because in nephrogenic diabetes insipidus, the problem in the kidney rather than a lack of ADH secretion.

Lithium-induced polyuria and diabetes insipidus: Treatment

Treatment algorithm

Let's outline a systematic approach to managing this problem based on a classic paper by Martin (1993).

Step 1. Change lithium to a single dose at bedtime. This gives time for the nephrons to recover before the next dose of lithium.

Step 2. Reduce the dose of lithium if possible

Step 3. Add potassium chloride 20 mEq per day (either by increasing foods rich in potassium or by giving a packet/tablet of potassium chloride)

Step 4. Add amiloride 10 mg/day. Amiloride is a potassium-sparing diuretic that is less likely to increase lithium levels that thiazide diuretics. However, we should be cautious. Increase to 10 mg twice daily if the 10 mg/day does not work.

Wouldn't adding a diuretic make polyuria worse? Lithium causes polyuria by blocking the effect of ADH in the distal and collecting tubule. Amiloride hinders the entrance of lithium into the tubule epithelium thus allowing ADH to exert its effect. Clinical response to amiloride usually occurs within one to two weeks. Amiloride is probably the medication of choice as it does not produce hypokalemia or profound volume depletion. However, it may cause serum levels of lithium to rise, though less than with the addition of hydrochlorothiazide.

Step 5. If that does not work, stop the amiloride and cautiously add hydrochlorothiazide 25 mg/day. Keep in mind that hydrochlorothiazide will increase the lithium level. So, strongly consider reducing the dose of the lithium at the same time that hydrochlorothiazide is added.

If needed increase hydrochlorothiazide to 25 mg twice daily.

Unlike amiloride, hydrochlorothiazide works by directly antagonizing ADH. Hydrochlorothiazide should be used with caution, as it can cause hypokalemia. Also, since it increases resorption of sodium and lithium in the proximal tubule, hydrochlorothiazide can lead to higher serum lithium levels. Thus, during concomitant use of hydrochlorothiazide with lithium, the patient must be monitored closely for toxicity and dehydration, and lithium levels should be drawn frequently when the diuretic is first added.

Step 6: If neither amiloride nor hydrochlorothiazide worked adequately, we can try them both together.

Step 7: Use indomethacin 50 mg three times a day. Indomethacin is an inhibitor of the prostaglandin system that may be involved in the development of lithium-induced diabetes insipidus. Caution is needed because it may increase lithium levels. The role of indomethacin in the algorithm is for patients who are resistant to the other treatments or who require a rapid reduction in polyuria for some reason.

URINARY HESITANCY/RETENTION

Urinary hesitancy or retention due to atomoxetine

Question: A male patient with ADHD developed urinary retention on atomoxetine. Are there any tricks to get around urinary retention caused by atomoxetine? The side effect started when the dose was pushed up to 60 mg daily. Atomoxetine 40 mg was helpful, but insufficient for fully treating inattention symptoms.

<u>Urinary hesitancy and retention</u>

When there is a delay between when a person decides to urinate and when urination actually starts, we call this "urinary hesitancy".

And, if the person tries to urinate but is unable to do so even though the bladder is full, we call this "urinary retention".

The two situations are related to each other—urinary hesitancy can be thought of as a milder version of the same problem that can lead to urinary retention. So, we can discuss the two conditions together.

How often does atomoxetine cause urinary hesitancy/ retention?

Many psychiatric medications can cause urinary hesitancy or retention; atomoxetine is one of them.

I was surprised to read in one publication the authors' assertion that with atomoxetine, "urinary side-effects are exceedingly rare" (Desarkar and Sinha, 2006). Let's see if that is true.

A simple way to estimate how often a medication is the cause of a particular problem is to take the percentage of patients on the medication who had that problem and subtract from it the percentage of patients on placebo who had that problem. This "placebo-subtracted" rate is an estimate of the percentage of cases in which the medication was causally related to the problem. Makes sense, right?

According to the Prescribing Information for atomoxetine (Strattera®), in placebo-controlled clinical trials for ADHD in adults, the rates for urinary hesitancy and retention were as follows (rounded off to the nearest 0.5%):

– Urinary hesitancy: atomoxetine 5.5%, placebo 0.5%; placebo-subtracted rate 5%. That's a lot!

– Urinary retention: atomoxetine 1.5%, placebo 0%; placebo-subtracted rate 1.5%. For a serious problem like urinary retention, that is also a lot!

Who? Who is more likely to get urinary retention on atomoxetine?

1. Poor metabolizers of CYP2D6

Atomoxetine is metabolized by cytochrome P450 2D6. Poor metabolizers of CYP2D6 are much more likely to get urinary retention on atomoxetine than extensive ("normal") metabolizers—6% versus 1% (Prescribing Information).

2. Presumably, being on a medication that inhibits CYP2D6

3. Higher dose

Like most side effects, urinary hesitancy/ retention associated with atomoxetine is dose-related. In the case noted above, the side effect started only after the dose was increased to 60 mg/day. Similarly, in a published case report, urinary retention occurred only after the dose was increased to 60 mg/day (Mutlu et al., 2015).

<u>When? How long after starting the atomoxetine?</u>

Urinary hesitancy or retention tends to occur very soon after the person is started on atomoxetine or the dose is increased. Here are some examples to show this:

– A 16-year-old boy who developed acute retention of urine three days after being started on atomoxetine 25 mg/day and needed to be catheterized (Desarkar and Sinha, 2006).

– In an 8-year-old boy, when atomoxetine was increased to 60 mg/day, urinary retention occurred the very first time he took the higher dose of 60 mg (Mutlu et al., 2015).

– A 12-year-old boy who was started on atomoxetine 25 mg/day developed urinary symptoms on the very first day and acute urinary retention on the second day (Sahin et al., 2015).

– A 41-year-old man who was on fluoxetine 20 mg per day "urgently" reported urinary hesitancy a week after being started on atomoxetine (Gandhi et al., 2017).

– A 7-year-old boy presented within the first week after starting on atomoxetine 18 mg/day with complaints of abdominal pain and difficulty urinating (Turan et al., 2020).

How to manage medication-induced urinary hesitancy/retention

No specific treatment has been reported for urinary hesitancy/ retention specifically due to atomoxetine. But, certain interventions have worked for urinary hesitancy/ retention due to other medications.

Many psychotropic medications have been associated with urinary hesitancy or retention. Urinary hesitancy/ retention occurs due to obstruction at the outlet from the urinary bladder (structural or due to the smooth muscle sphincter not relaxing open) and/or due to the bladder wall not contracting normally.

What are our options if urinary hesitancy/ retention occurs due to a psychotropic medication? Of course, urinary retention due to medication may be an emergency, and catheterization of the bladder may be needed. What then?

Stop the medication

Stopping the medication that caused the problem tends to resolve the problem. For example, in all the published case reports that I reviewed, atomoxetine-induced urinary hesitancy/ retention quickly went away once the atomoxetine was stopped.

Lower the dose, if possible

Like most side effects, medication-induced urinary hesitancy is dose-dependent. So, if reducing the dose is an option, this may relieve the problem in some patients.

Eliminate, if possible, any contributory factors

– Enlarged prostate

– Medications with anticholinergic activity

– Medications with sympathomimetic activity

But, what if we want to continue on the psychiatric medication that is causing the patient's urinary hesitancy/ retention because it is important and valuable for the patient? Is there anything that we can do to treat the urinary hesitancy/ retention?

A person can urinate if there is enough cholinergic activity (e.g., allowing the bladder to contract properly) and the noradrenergic activity is not too high, because that causes the

The intervention will depend on whether the urinary hesitancy is due to:

– Increased noradrenergic effect

– Anticholinergic activity.

Let's look at what we might do in each of these two scenarios.

Add a selective alpha-1a receptor blocker?

Psychiatric medications that strongly inhibit norepinephrine reuptake are believed to be associated with a higher risk of urinary hesitancy/ retention (Asnis et al., 2016).

This is believed to be because norepinephrine stimulates the alpha-1 receptors that are present in the bladder sphincter and make the sphincter contract, closing off the outlet from the bladder.

– In two case series, eight (Kasper and Wolf, 2002) and six (Demyttenaere et al., 2001) patients with urinary hesitancy due to reboxetine were treated with tamsulosin (a selective alpha-1a receptor blocker), which relieved the problem quickly, within 20 minutes (Kasper and Wolf, 2002). Note: Reboxetine is a selective norepinephrine reuptake inhibitor (like atomoxetine), which is not available in the US but is available in many other countries.

– Two patients with painful ejaculation and urinary hesitancy due to reboxetine were successfully treated with tamsulosin, which quickly resolved these side effects (Demyttenaere and Huygens, 2002).

– Two patients with urinary hesitancy due to levomilnacipran were successfully treated with tamsulosin so that the antidepressant did not have to be stopped (Asnis et al., 2016).

Note: Only a medication that is selective for blocking alpha-1a receptors that are present in the urinary tract should be considered. Using a non-selective medication that blocks alpha-1 receptors everywhere (e.g., terazosin, prazosin, doxazosin) carries a risk of hypotension. Also, those medications need to be titrated up over many days or weeks while urinary hesitancy/ retention is an urgent problem.

Note: Even though tamsulosin was used in the case series/ case reports noted above, it is not the only selective alpha-1a receptor blocker available. The following three are available in the US and all three are generic and inexpensive; they are listed here in alphabetical order:

1. Alfuzosin (brand name Uroxatral®)

2. Silodosin (brand name Rapaflo®)

3. Tamsulosin (brand name Flomax)

<u>Add bethanechol?</u>

Bethanechol stimulates muscarinic cholinergic receptors. So, at times, it is used when the anticholinergic effects of another medication need to be counteracted. Due to its cholinergic activity, bethanechol stimulates motility of the gastrointestinal tract and stimulates the urinary bladder to contract.

For example, in a case report, bethanechol was effective in treating urinary retention due to olanzapine (Greco et al., 2019).

In other situations, it may be appropriate to increase bladder contraction by using bethanechol. Bethanechol (generic and brand name Urecholine®) selectively stimulates muscarinic cholinergic receptors. So, at times, it is used when the anticholinergic effects of another medication need to be counteracted. Due to its cholinergic activity, bethanechol stimulates motility of the gastrointestinal tract and stimulates the urinary bladder to contract.

On a personal note, when I had an appendicectomy many years ago, I had persistent, complete urinary retention postoperatively, which required repeated catheterization. When the surgical team came on rounds, I asked them to give me bethanechol and explained how it works. Even though bethanechol has an FDA indication for "acute postoperative and postpartum nonobstructive (functional) urinary retention and for neurogenic atony of the urinary bladder with retention" (source: Bethanechol Prescribing Information), the treatment team didn't seem to be aware of this option. But, since they knew I was a physician, they agreed to prescribe it. Within a short time, bethanechol completely resolved the problem that had been so troublesome and had kept me in the hospital unnecessarily!

Now, let's look at some examples of using bethanechol to treat urinary hesitancy or retention due to a psychotropic medication.

– In a case report, bethanechol was effective in completely resolving urinary retention that was attributed to olanzapine (Greco et al., 2019). It was started at 10 mg three times a day and later increased to 10 mg three times a day plus 20 mg at bedtime. In case you are wondering, urinary retention associated with the use of olanzapine has reported by others as well (e.g., Mirzakhani et al., 2020; Cohen et al., 2007; Semaan et al., 2006).

– Two cases were reported of urinary hesitancy associated with buprenorphine treatment that was successfully treated in both of them with bethanechol 25 mg up to twice a day (Varma et al., 2011).

References

Allen HM, Jackson RL, Winchester MD, Deck LV, Allon M. Indomethacin in the treatment of lithium-induced nephrogenic diabetes insipidus. Arch Intern Med 1989;149(5):1123-6.

Asnis GM, Caneva E, Henderson MA. A review of antidepressant-induced urinary hesitancy: a focus on levomilnacipran ER including two case presentations(5633). Expert Opin Drug Saf. 2016 May;15(5):717-25. doi: 10.1517/14740338.2016.1164138. Epub 2016 Apr 1. PMID: 26967743.

Ball S, McCullough J. Diabetes Insipidus. 2015 Apr 12. In: De Groot LJ, Chrousos G, Dungan K, Feingold KR, Grossman A, Hershman JM, Koch C, Korbonits M, McLachlan R, New M, Purnell J, Rebar R, Singer F, Vinik A, editors. Endotext [Internet]. South Dartmouth (MA): MDText.com, Inc.; 2000-. Available from   http://www.ncbi.nlm.nih.gov/books/NBK279011/   PubMed   PMID: 25905242.

Batlle DC, von Riotte AB, Gaviria M, Grupp M. Amelioration of polyuria by amiloride in patients receiving long-term lithium therapy. N Engl J Med. 1985;312(7):408-14.

Bedford JJ, Weggery S, Ellis G, McDonald FJ, Joyce PR, Leader JP, Walker RJ. Lithium-induced nephrogenic diabetes insipidus: renal effects of amiloride. Clin J Am Soc Nephrol. 2008 Sep;3(5):1324-31. PubMed PMID: 18596116; PubMed Central PMCID: PMC2518801.

Behl T, Kotwani A, Kaur I, Goel H. Mechanisms of prolonged lithium therapy-induced nephrogenic diabetes insipidus. Eur J Pharmacol. 2015 May 15;755:27-33. PubMed PMID: 25746463.

Bendz H, Aurell M. Drug-induced diabetes insipidus: incidence, prevention and management. Drug Saf. 1999;21(6):449-56.

Bichet DG. Nephrogenic diabetes insipidus. Adv Chronic Kidney Dis. 2006 Apr;13(2):96-104. Review. PubMed PMID: 16580609.

Bockenhauer D, Bichet DG. Pathophysiology, diagnosis and management of nephrogenic diabetes insipidus. Nat Rev Nephrol. 2015 Oct;11(10):576-88. PubMed PMID: 26077742.

Camporeale A, Day KA, Ruff D, Arsenault J, Williams D, Kelsey DK. Profile of sexual and genitourinary treatment-emergent adverse events associated with atomoxetine treatment: a pooled analysis. Drug Saf. 2013 Aug;36(8):663-71. doi: 10.1007/s40264-013-0074-2. PMID: 23775507.

Corbin Bush N, Twombley K, Ahn J, Oliveira C, Arnold S, Maalouf NM, Sakhaee K. Prevalence and spot urine risk factors for renal stones in children taking topiramate.   J   Pediatr   Urol.   2013   Dec;9(6   Pt   A):884-9.   doi: 10.1016/j.jpurol.2012.12.005. Epub 2013 Feb 1. PubMed PMID: 23375465;

PubMed Central PMCID: PMC3644535.

Danuser H, Bemis K, Thor KB. Pharmacological analysis of the noradrenergic control of central sympathetic and somatic reflexes controlling the lower urinary tract in the anesthetized cat. J Pharmacol Exp Ther. 1995 Aug;274(2):820-5. PMID: 7636745.

de Groot T, Sinke AP, Kortenoeven ML, Alsady M, Baumgarten R, Devuyst O, Loffing J, Wetzels JF, Deen PM. Acetazolamide Attenuates Lithium-Induced Nephrogenic Diabetes Insipidus. J Am Soc Nephrol. 2016 Jul;27(7):2082-91. PubMed PMID: 26574046; PubMed Central PMCID: PMC4926986.

Demyttenaere K, Huygens R, Van Buggenhout R. Tamsulosin as an effective treatment for reboxetine-associated urinary hesitancy. Int Clin Psychopharmacol. 2001 Nov;16(6):353-5. doi: 10.1097/00004850-200111000-00006. PMID: 11712624.

Demyttenaere K, Huygens R. Painful ejaculation and urinary hesitancy in association with antidepressant therapy: relief with tamsulosin. Eur Neuropsychopharmacol. 2002 Aug;12(4):337-41. doi: 10.1016/s0924-977x(02)00040-8. PMID: 12126873.

Desarkar P, Sinha VK. Acute urinary retention associated with atomoxetine use. Aust N Z J Psychiatry. 2006 Oct;40(10):936. doi: 10.1080/j.1440-1614.2006.01914.x. PMID: 16959021.

Devuyst O. Physiopathology and diagnosis of nephrogenic diabetes insipidus. Ann Endocrinol (Paris). 2012 Apr;73(2):128-9. PubMed PMID: 22503803.

Fenske W, Allolio B. Clinical review: Current state and future perspectives in the diagnosis of diabetes insipidus: a clinical review. J Clin Endocrinol Metab. 2012 Oct;97(10):3426-37. PubMed PMID: 22855338.

Finch CK, Kelley KW, Williams RB. Treatment of lithium-induced diabetes insipidus with amiloride. Pharmacotherapy. 2003;23(4):546-50.

Gandhi R, Narang P, Lippmann S. Urinary Hesitancy Associated With Atomoxetine. Prim Care Companion CNS Disord. 2017 Sep 14;19(5):17l02095. doi: 10.4088/PCC.17l02095. PMID: 28930379.

Gitlin M. Lithium and the kidney: an updated review. Drug Saf. 1999;20(3):231-43.

Gordon CE, Vantzelfde S, Francis JM. Acetazolamide in Lithium-Induced Nephrogenic Diabetes Insipidus. N Engl J Med. 2016 Nov 17;375(20):2008-2009. PubMed PMID: 27959610.

Greco FA, Simms NJ, Athappilly GK. Bethanechol as a Corrective for Urinary Retention Associated With Olanzapine Administration. Prim Care Companion CNS Disord. 2019 Oct 31;21(5):19l02429. doi: 10.4088/PCC.19l02429. PMID: 31682336.

Jion YI, Raff A, Grosberg BM, Evans RW. The risk and management of kidney stones from the use of topiramate and zonisamide in migraine and idiopathic intracranial hypertension. Headache. 2015 Jan;55(1):161-6. doi: 10.1111/head.12480. Epub 2014 Dec 9. Review. PubMed PMID: 25486999.

Kasper S, Wolf R. Successful treatment of reboxetine-induced urinary hesitancy with tamsulosin. Eur Neuropsychopharmacol. 2002 Apr;12(2):119-22. doi: 10.1016/s0924-977x(01)00144-4. PMID: 11872327.

Kasper S. Managing reboxetine-associated urinary hesitancy in a patient with major depressive disorder: a case study. Psychopharmacology (Berl). 2002 Feb;159(4):445-6. doi: 10.1007/s00213-001-0971-4. Epub 2001 Dec 20. PMID: 11823898.

Khanna A. Acquired nephrogenic diabetes insipidus. Semin Nephrol. 2006 May;26(3):244-8. PubMed PMID: 16713497.

Knoers N. Nephrogenic Diabetes Insipidus. 2000 Feb 12 [updated 2012 Jun 14]. In: Pagon RA, Adam MP, Ardinger HH, Wallace SE, Amemiya A, Bean LJH, Bird TD, Ledbetter N, Mefford HC, Smith RJH, Stephens K, editors. GeneReviews® [Internet]. Seattle (WA): University of Washington, Seattle; 1993-2017. Available from http://www.ncbi.nlm.nih.gov/books/NBK1177/ PubMed PMID: 20301356.

Kosten TR, Forrest JN. Treatment of severe lithium-induced polyuria with amiloride. Am J Psychiatry. 1986;143(12):1563-8.

Leroy C, Karrouz W, Douillard C, Do Cao C, Cortet C, Wémeau JL, Vantyghem MC. Diabetes insipidus. Ann Endocrinol (Paris). 2013 Dec;74(5-6):496-507. PubMed PMID: 24286605.

Majzoub JA, Srivatsa A. Diabetes insipidus: clinical and basic aspects. Pediatr Endocrinol Rev. 2006 Dec;4 Suppl 1:60-5. PubMed PMID: 17261971.

Makaryus AN, McFarlane SI. Diabetes insipidus: diagnosis and treatment of a complex disease. Cleve Clin J Med. 2006 Jan;73(1):65-71. PubMed PMID: 16444918.

Marmura MJ. Safety of topiramate for treating migraines. Expert Opin Drug Saf. 2014 Sep;13(9):1241-7. doi: 10.1517/14740338.2014.934669. Epub 2014 Aug 6. PMID: 25096056.

Martin A. Clinical management of lithium-induced polyuria. Hosp Community Psychiatry. 1993;44(5):427-8.

McGrane IR, Campbell TJ. Probable Genitourinary Adverse Events Associated With Atomoxetine in an Adult Male: A Case Report. J Pharm Pract. 2020 Aug 31:897190020953022. doi: 10.1177/0897190020953022. Epub ahead of print. PMID: 32862763.

Mutlu C, Yorbik O, Ipek H, Tanju IA. Acute Urinary Retention Associated with Increased Dose of Atomoxetine in a Child: A Case Report. Klinik Psikofarmakoloji Bülteni-Bulletin of Clinical Psychopharmacology. 2015:25:3, 299-301, DOI: 10.5455/bcp.20140408015727. *Not on PubMed.*

Raedler TJ. Will lithium damage my kidneys? J Psychiatry Neurosci. 2012 May;37(3):E5-6. PubMed PMID: 22515988; PubMed Central PMCID: PMC3341412.

Rej S, Segal M, Low NC, Mucsi I, Holcroft C, Shulman K, Looper K. The McGill Geriatric Lithium-Induced Diabetes Insipidus Clinical Study (McGLIDICS). Can J Psychiatry. 2014 Jun;59(6):327-34. PubMed PMID: 25007407; PubMed Central PMCID: PMC4079152.

Robertson GL. Diabetes insipidus: Differential diagnosis and management. Best Pract Res Clin Endocrinol Metab. 2016 Mar;30(2):205-18. PubMed PMID: 27156759.

Sands JM, Bichet DG; American College of Physicians.; American Physiological Society.. Nephrogenic diabetes insipidus. Ann Intern Med. 2006 Feb 7;144(3):186-94. PubMed PMID: 16461963.

Topamax Prescribing Information. Available at: http://www.janssenlabels.com/package-insert/product-monograph/prescribing-information/TOPAMAX-pi.pdf. Accessed on May 17, 2020.

Tredget J, Kirov A, Kirov G. Effects of chronic lithium treatment on renal function. J Affect Disord. 2010 Nov;126(3):436-40. PubMed PMID: 20483164.

Trepiccione F, Christensen BM. Lithium-induced nephrogenic diabetes insipidus: new clinical and experimental findings. J Nephrol. 2010 Nov-Dec;23 Suppl 16:S43-8. PubMed PMID: 21170888.

Whiskey E, Taylor D. A review of the adverse effects and safety of noradrenergic antidepressants. J Psychopharmacol. 2013 Aug;27(8):732-9. doi: 10.1177/0269881113492027. Epub 2013 Jun 19. PMID: 23784737.

CHAPTER 18: WEIGHT

WEIGHT GAIN

Does weight gain with second-generation (atypical) antipsychotics plateau after the first few months?

Weight gain and related metabolic side effects are a huge problem in people prescribed second-generation (atypical) antipsychotics. Among these medications, olanzapine and clozapine are associated with the greatest probability and amount of weight gain.

A very important question to consider in the risk-benefit analysis is whether the weight gain will stop (plateau) after some time or whether it is likely that patients will continue to gain weight for many months or years if they keep taking the medication.

Some people believe that weight gain with these medications tends to plateau after just a few months. Is this true or is it just wishful thinking?

Study no. 1

A large but retrospective study (Osborn et al., 2018) looked at weight gain with olanzapine, quetiapine, and risperidone in several thousands of patients in "real-life" clinical settings who were followed for two years.

– With all three medications, the weight gain continued to increase over the two-year follow up since first starting the medication.

– Patients who were prescribed olanzapine tended to be ones with lower weight at baseline.

– Patients prescribed olanzapine gained more weight than those on either quetiapine or risperidone during the first six months as well as during the rest of the two years.

– This remained true even after statistical adjustment for the lower baseline weight in patients who were prescribed olanzapine.

Study no. 2

Another retrospective study looked at weight gain in thousands of patients in "real-life" clinical settings who took an oral or depot antipsychotic for three years (Bushe et al., 2012).

– For all the antipsychotics, weight gain was more rapid during the first six months.

– After the first six months, the weight gain was slower but did not plateau.

Study no. 3

Next, let's look at a study from the manufacturer of olanzapine (Kinon et al., 2001). The abstract states that the study found that in patients followed for three years, weight gain on olanzapine plateaued after 39 weeks (roughly 9 months).

But, if we read the paper, we see that this was true only for those patients who continued to take olanzapine for three years. Out of about 1300 patients who started on olanzapine, 573 patients took it for at least 39 weeks, 293 took it for at least 2.5 years, and only 147 took it for the full three years of follow up. The statement that weight gain plateaued ignores the fact that patients were continually discontinuing the olanzapine as time went on. In my opinion, it is not far-fetched to speculate that patients whose weight gain plateaued were more willing to continue taking the olanzapine while those whose weight gain did not plateau stopped taking it.

Bottom line

- Weight gain due to second-generation antipsychotics is clearly most rapid in the first six months.

- After the first six to nine months, the rate of weight gain tends to slow.

- For some patients, weight gain may plateau after some time, but in others, it may continue to increase even after two to three years!

- So, the idea that weight does not continue to increase after the first few months on a second-generation antipsychotic, which I have heard several times, is part of psychopharMYTHology.

We cannot give our patients false reassurance in this regard.

Predictors of medication-induced weight gain

Do adolescents have more metabolic side effects with second-generation antipsychotics?

It is concerning that olanzapine continues to be prescribed to many children and adolescents, especially on the inpatient units. In talking to other clinicians, I am finding that those who work on an inpatient unit seem to be more likely to prescribe olanzapine when a second-generation antipsychotic is needed. But, it is the outpatient psychiatrists who have to deal with the weight gain and other metabolic side effects that occur over the longer-term. All clinicians should take both the short-term and long-term perspective in choosing from among the second-generation antipsychotics.

In this section, I want to answer the question of whether adolescents are more likely than adults to have metabolic side effects with second-generation antipsychotics and whether these side effects are more severe in adolescents. I hope that clinicians will keep these issues in mind and discuss them as part of informed consent.

One paper (Kryzhanovskaya et al., 2012) compared adolescent and adult patients who had taken olanzapine for at least 24 weeks. It compared the incidence of weight gain and other metabolic side effects between adolescents (about 180) and in adults (about 4300).

The findings

Mean weight gain during olanzapine treatment: adolescents–about 25 pounds; adults–about 10.5 pounds. This difference was statistically significant. Note that 25 pounds was the mean weight gain in these adolescents, so many patients gained more than that.

Percentage with clinically significant weight gain since starting the olanzapine (7% of baseline weight or more)—Are you ready for this?—adolescents 89% (89% had clinically significant weight gain!); adults, 55%.

Percentage who went from normal blood sugar to abnormally increased blood sugar—adolescents 9%; adults 1%.

Methodological tip for clinicians

Whenever we read about any study, we should think—Does the kind of patients who were included in the study suggest that the findings of the study may be an underestimate of the facts or an overestimation?

In this study (Kryzhanovskaya et al., 2012), only patients who had taken olanzapine for at least two years were included. Would you agree that we may expect that some of the patients who had the worst weight gain or who developed increased blood sugar after starting olanzapine may have discontinued the medication before they had been on it for two years or more?

If so, this study is more likely to have underestimated rather than overestimated the weight gain and metabolic side effects of olanzapine.

Bottom line

The concern about clinically-significant weight gain and other metabolic side effects is even greater in adolescents than in adults.

All medications can cause some side effects, but we must take into consideration what percentage of them had a particular side effect and how significant and persistent the side effect was.

In the case of olanzapine prescribed to adolescents, the amount of weight gain is substantial and it occurs in an astronomically high percentage of them (89% in this study).

This information should be taken into account while recommending a second-generation antipsychotic in an adolescent patient.

Also, this information is important to share as part of informed consent.

HTR2C polymorphisms and medication-induced weight gain

Weight gain is one of the most problematic side effects of second-generation (atypical) antipsychotics. Clinicians who prescribe these medications note that some patients seem to have marked weight gain on a particular medication while others have little or no weight gain on the same medication. Why?

Regulation of appetite/weight is complex with many biological mechanisms involved. So, not surprisingly, there is a long list of genetic variations that have been evaluated with regard to antipsychotic-induced weight gain. One of the most important ones of these is a polymorphism of the serotonin 2C receptor.

5-HT2C receptor and appetite/weight

The serotonin 2C (5-HT2C) receptor is involved in regulation of appetite and weight. In addition to histamine H1 receptor blockade, effects at 5-HT2C receptors are believed to be related to antipsychotic-induced weight gain.

– The 5-HT2C receptor gene (HTR2C) is expressed in the hypothalamus, including the paraventricular nucleus, which is important in weight regulation (Correll and Malhotra, 2004).

– Mice in whom the 5-HT2C receptor gene is "knocked out," have chronic hyperphagia and obesity (Tecott et al., 1995).

– The 5-HT2C receptor interacts with the signaling pathways for melanocortin and leptin (MacNeil and Müller, 2016), which are involved in the regulation of appetite and weight

-759C/T polymorphism of HTR2C

The gene that codes for the 5-HT2C receptor is called HTR2C.

One polymorphism of HTR2C is -759C/T which means that in position -759 of the gene (which is in its promoter region), the normal C (cytosine) is replaced by a T (thymine). This polymorphism's number is rs3813929. This is the polymorphism that is tested for in the commercially available Genomind® assay when they say "5-HT2C receptor".

This polymorphism has been associated with obesity and type II diabetes in normal subjects (Gressier et al., 2016).

The T allele, which is less common than the C allele, is protective against antipsychotic weight gain (Reynolds, 2012).

This association is present in the case of both antipsychotics with high affinity (e.g., clozapine, olanzapine) and relatively low affinity (e.g., risperidone) to the 5-HT2C receptor (Reynolds, 2012).

One of the first studies was done in 123 Han Chinese patients who were drug-naive prior to entering the study (Reynolds et al., 2002). While 28% of the subjects without the T allele gained a significant amount of weight (7% or more of their baseline body weight), none of those with the T allele had significant weight gain.

Note: Some negative studies on this association included participants with extensive prior treatment with antipsychotics, which limits their utility.

Studies that found an association: Reynolds et al. (2002), Reynolds et al. (2003), Miller et al. (2005), Laika et al. (2010), Hoekstra et al. (2010), Opgen-Rhein et al. (2010), Gregoor et al. (2010).

Studies that did not find an association: Basile et al. (2001), Tsai et al. (2001), Park et al. (2008), Gunes et al. (2009), Correia et al. (2010), Sicard et al. (2010), Thompson et al. (2010), Gregoor et al. (2011), Kuzman et al. (2011), Kang et al. (2011), Houston et al. (2012), Del Castillo et al. (2013), Kang et al. (2014), Ma et al. (2014), Grădinaru et al. (2017).

rs1414334 (C/G) polymorphism of HTR2C

Those with the C allele are at higher risk of antipsychotic-induced weight gain (MacNeil and Müller, 2016).

So, just as for the -759C/T polymorphism, the minor (less common) allele is protective against antipsychotic-induced weight gain.

Monitoring

Monitoring for metabolic side effects in patients on a second-generation (atypical) antipsychotic

What clinical measurements and laboratory tests should be done in adult patients on second-generation antipsychotics to monitor them for possible development of metabolic side effects?

When and how often should these evaluations be done?

A small number clinicians test more frequently than is needed but, unfortunately, the majority do these evaluations less often than is recommended (or not at all; Mitchell et al., 2012; Weisman et al., 2012; Dhamane et al., 2013).

Who decides?

The key guideline on this issue of how to monitor adult patients who are on a second-generation ("atypical") antipsychotic for metabolic syndrome is still the classic paper published in 2004 from a consensus development conference of several leading professional organizations. The full text of this article is available free at this link:

http://care.diabetesjournals.org/content/27/2/596.full.pdf

But, I will summarize the main points here for you.

What should be monitored and how often?

The consensus conference guidelines recommend monitoring of the following with regard to potential metabolic side effects of second-generation antipsychotics.

Different aspects of the monitoring should be done at Baseline, 4 weeks, 8 weeks, every 3 months, once a year, and every 5 years.

According to the Consensus guideline, all of the following should be done at Baseline. Then, after starting the second-generation antipsychotic:

-   Personal/family history: Annually

- Weight (BMI): At 4 weeks, 8 weeks, 12 weeks, and then quarterly

- Waist circumference: Annually

- Blood pressure: At 12 weeks and then annually

- Fasting plasma glucose: At 12 weeks and then annually

- Fasting lipid profile: At 12 weeks and then every 5 years

Notes:

– This is the minimum monitoring they recommended.

– Of course, if a significant change and/or abnormality is found, the frequency of monitoring should be increased.

– Obviously, it does not matter who does the monitoring. For example, it may be the primary care physician who is measuring some or all of these things. But, we cannot rely on the primary care physician because it is very unlikely that they will measure some of these things at the frequencies recommended above. If we are prescribing the second-generation antipsychotic, ultimately we must make sure that this monitoring is being done.

– One important criticism that I have of this guideline is that it recommends the same monitoring for all the second-generation antipsychotics irrespective if they carry a low, medium, or high risk of metabolic side effects. Does it make sense to do metabolic monitoring with equal intensity in patients on lower-risk medications like aripiprazole or ziprasidone and patients on higher risk medications like olanzapine?

– Also, I have bad news–publication of this consensus guideline does not seem to have significantly improved the prevalence of metabolic monitoring in patients on second-generation antipsychotics (Dhamane et al., 2012). So, we'll have to think harder about how to improve the situation.

Comments on measuring weight circumference

Measuring the waist circumference is important and measuring the weight alone is not enough. This is because visceral fat is bad metabolically.

But, measuring waist circumference requires a specific method and is not done by simply putting a tape measure around the patient's waist.

Some thoughts about weight circumference:

Also, in mental health practice, to be frank, it is awkward to put your arms around the patient's waist to measure the patient's waist circumference. I know that we are medical professionals and I am not saying that we should not measure waist circumference. I am just acknowledging something that is a fact.

If the patient is not overweight, is there any need to measure the waist circumference at baseline?

Similarly, if the weight has not shown a significant increase, is there any need to check or recheck waist circumference annually?

Monitoring for metabolic side effects in children and adolescents on a second-generation (atypical) antipsychotic

The American Academy of Child and Adolescent Psychiatry has developed a Clinical Practice Guideline on Antipsychotic Medication but this is pending review by the AHRQ and has not been published.

In the meanwhile, we can look to our Northern neighbors for guidance. The Canadian Alliance for Monitoring Effectiveness and Safety of Antipsychotics in Children (CAMESA) published evidence-based recommendations for monitoring safety of second-generation antipsychotics in children and youth (Pringsheim et al., 2011). The full text of the paper is available free at https://www.ncbi.nlm.nih.gov/pmc/articles/PMC3143700/. Note that this guideline is more than five years old, but the guideline for adults is even older.

The guidelines and monitoring forms for specific antipsychotics are available free at http://camesaguideline.org

Is waist circumference relevant in children?

Based on a systematic review of primary studies, "strong" evidence was found, that waist circumference is important to measure in children and adolescents on (alphabetically) aripiprazole, olanzapine, quetiapine, and risperidone (Pringsheim et al., 2011). The evidence for recommending that waist circumference should be measured for children on clozapine or ziprasidone was judged to be "weak" (Pringsheim et al., 2011).

For example, for children on risperidone, measurement of waist circumference is recommended by the CAMESA guideline at baseline, 1 month, 2 months, 3 months, 6 months, 9 months, and 12 months.

Also, this change can occur within just four weeks of starting on the second-generation antipsychotic. In children and youth 4 to 19 years old who had not taken an antipsychotic in the past, there was a statistically significant increase in waist circumference after only four weeks of treatment with olanzapine, quetiapine, or risperidone (Correll et al., 2009). The average increase in waist circumference after four weeks was about 3 cm with quetiapine and risperidone and about 4 cm with olanzapine.

Is measuring BMI at four weeks useful?

The guideline (Pringsheim et al., 2011) specifically noted that significant changes in weight and waist circumference can occur in children within four weeks of starting a second-generation antipsychotic (Correll et al., 2009).

After four weeks of treatment, statistically significant increases in BMI were found in patients treated with any of the four second-generation antipsychotics used in the study: aripiprazole, olanzapine, quetiapine, and risperidone (Correll et al., 2009).

The mean increase in BMI after four weeks of treatment, as a percentage of the BMI at baseline, was aripiprazole 3%, olanzapine 8%, quetiapine 4.5%, and risperidone 5% (Correll et al., 2009).

This is why the CAMESA guidelines recommend that the measurement of BMI should start early in treatment. As an example, for children and adolescents taking risperidone, the CAMESA guidelines recommend measurement of body mass index (BMI) at baseline, 1 month, 2 months, 3 months, 6 months, 9 months, and 12 months.

Management of medication-induced weight gain

1. Metformin

Metformin is currently one of the most important pharmacological treatments for metabolic adverse effects of antipsychotics. Those of us who prescribe antipsychotic medications must learn about how and when to prescribe metformin. I think only a small percentage of people in whom metformin might be a good option are currently being prescribed metformin by us.

In a meta-analysis of various treatments for antipsychotic-induced weight gain and metabolic abnormalities, metformin was the most effective of all of them (Maayan et al., 2010). Of course, none of them was tremendously effective. But the average weight loss with metformin was slightly greater even than that for topiramate.

Also, as discussed below, metformin is a good choice because it not only helps to reduce weight but also improves other aspects of the metabolic profile like glucose and lipids. It works not only by appetite suppression but also by several other mechanisms (see below).

How does it work?

There are two practical reasons why we may want to know how metformin works.

1. Firstly, it may seem odd to give a diabetes medication if the blood sugar is normal and we may worry that it will drop the blood sugar. But actually, since metformin does not increase the release of insulin and it only partially reduced gluconeogenesis in the liver, it is rare for hypoglycemia to occur (Kirpichnikov et al., 2002).

If it doesn't increase insulin secretion, then how does it work? There are multiple mechanisms and some of these are only recently being understood. Metformin can help with reducing weight, glucose, and lipids by:

– Blocking production of glucose in the liver (Kirpichnikov et al., 2002)

– Increasing peripheral insulin sensitivity (Kirpichnikov et al., 2002)

– Reducing the increased appetite that antipsychotics cause due to their effects on the brain

– Slowing of gastric emptying due to stimulating secretion of glucagon-like peptide-1 (Mannucci et al., 2004)

– Possibly affecting activity of hormones and neurotransmitters related to hunger and satiety (ghrelin, leptin, neuropeptide Y)

2. So, the second practical point, the significance of these multiple mechanisms of action, is that metformin works in our patients whether or not they have increased blood sugar and whether or not they have increased appetite. I'll repeat–metformin, an antidiabetic medication, should be considered even if the hemoglobin A1C is completely normal.

Does it work?

Yes — in some people and to some extent.

In a meta-analysis, metformin was found to be effective for improvement in body weight, body mass index, fasting glucose, fasting insulin, triglycerides, and total cholesterol in persons being treated with an antipsychotic medication (Zheng et al., 2015).

However, different parameters–weight, hemoglobin A1C, LDL cholesterol, triglycerides, fasting insulin–may improve in different persons.

(The benefit of metformin was also found in a later meta-analysis by de Silva et al., 2016)

In one study, of persons on clozapine, 29% lost 7% or more of their body weight (Chen et al., 2013).

Note: the weight tends to return to baseline if metformin is stopped (Chen et al., 2013).

How much is the benefit?

In combining multiple studies, the average weight loss was about 3 Kg or about 6.5 lbs (Maayan et al., 2010). Of course, "average" means that some patients will loose less than 3 Kg and some will loose more.

So it is important for us to know who is more likely to benefit from metformin.

Is the benefit sustained?

However, whether the benefits of metformin are sustained beyond 3 to 4 months is not clear from the clinical trials.

Who is more likely to benefit from metformin?

Who would be most likely to benefit from the addition of metformin for the management of weight gain or other metabolic adverse effects on an antipsychotic? While metformin should at least be considered in any such person, some are more likely to benefit from the addition of metformin.

Patient characteristics

1. Younger patients (e.g., younger than in their mid-4os in the Jarskog et al. (2013) study. This advantage in younger patients has repeatedly been shown. On the other hand, metformin is much less likely to effective in persons who have had chronic treatment with antipsychotics. So, this is important— let's not wait (weight?) for years before starting metformin!

2. Relatively recently been started on an antipsychotic (Hasnain and Vieweg, 2013). This overlaps with the first point above.

3. Overweight but not markedly obese (BMI less than 33 in the Jarskog et al., 2013 study)

4. Had rapid weight gain and/or increased glucose (Hasnain and Vieweg, 2013)

5. Non-smokers (Jarskog et al., 2013). Unclear why — the authors speculated that it may be because smoking already suppresses appetite.

Treatment characteristics

When the maintenance dose of metformin is higher (in the Zheng et al., 2015 meta-analysis, greater than 750 mg/day, but probably higher than that is better). This is also an important point. Often, clinicians prescribe metformin in too low a dose.

Metformin for antipsychotic-induced weight gain in children and adolescents?

Note: Metformin is FDA-approved for the treatment of type 2 diabetes mellitus in children 10 years or older. But, here, we are talking about the off-label treatment of weight gain in children and adolescents in whom the blood sugar is NOT elevated.

What did randomized, controlled trials find

Two randomized, controlled clinical trials have been published (Klein et al., 2006; Anagnostou et al., 2016) and a third RCT (Reeves et al., 2013) has been completed but its full results have not been published, though some data have been posted online and the full paper is under review.

All three randomized, controlled trials did find metformin to be more effective than placebo in children and adolescents for mitigating antipsychotic-induced weight gain.

How to dose metformin in children and adolescents

In children 6 to 9 years old, metformin may be started at 250 mg once daily after the largest meal of the day (Anagnostou et al., 2016). After one week, it can be increased to 250 mg twice daily and, if it is being tolerated, it can be increased to 500 mg twice daily after another week.

In patients 10 to 17 years old, metformin may be started at 500 mg once daily after the largest meal of the day (Klein et al., 2006; Anagnostou et al., 2016). After one week, we can increase to 500 mg twice daily and, if it is being tolerated, it may be increased to 850 mg twice daily after another week.

In one clinical trial (Reeves et al., 2013) in youth 8 to 19 years old, metformin was titrated up to the following doses:

< 50 Kg: 500 mg twice daily

50 to 70 Kg: 500 mg in the morning and 1000 mg in the evening

> 70 Kg: 1000 mg twice daily

Other important tips on using metformin

1. Before we even treat with metformin, we should consider the possibility of stopping the antipsychotic or, if applicable changing to one with a lower potential for weight gain, e.g., aripiprazole.

2. Evaluation of the outcome has to take into account the fact that children and adolescents are growing. So, when assessing the benefit of any intervention for antipsychotic-induced weight gain in children and adolescents, body mass index is more useful than body weight as the outcome measure we should look at.

3. The benefits of metformin typically become clear after several weeks of treatment, so a trial of metformin should last no less than 12 weeks, preferably more. The two published randomized, controlled trials discussed above lasted for 16 weeks and the third (unpublished) one lasted for 24 weeks.

4. In addition to metformin, counseling about diet and exercise must also be done, as was done in all three of the clinical trials. But, if the antipsychotic is being used to treat irritability in a patient with autism spectrum disorder, it may be hard to withhold high-calorie food since this may make the child even more irritable (McDougle, 2016).

Potential adverse effects of metformin

In an excellent paper published in 2016, Dr. Chittaranjan Andrade highlighted important safety issues related to the use of metformin to treat metabolic adverse effects of antipsychotic medications. Here, I recommend action items from his paper and from other relevant studies on the topic.

Gastrointestinal

The commonest adverse effects of metformin are abdominal discomfort, nausea, vomiting, diarrhea, or flatulence.

For example, in a meta-analysis of studies of metformin in the treatment of metabolic adverse effects of antipsychotics, the most common adverse effects were nausea/vomiting in 14% of patients and diarrhea in 7% of patients.

To prevent and treat gastrointestinal adverse effects, it is recommended

(Kirpichnikov et al., 2002; Andrade, 2016) that we should:

1. Prescribe extended-release metformin only

2. Ask the patient to take the metformin with meals

3. Titrate the dose up slowly

4. Reassure the patient that the gastrointestinal adverse effects tend to go away in about two to three weeks

5. If needed, temporarily reduce the dose. The gastrointestinal adverse effects, like most adverse effects, are dose related.

About 5% of persons cannot tolerate metformin due to gastrointestinal adverse effects (Kirpichnikov et al., 2002).

Vitamin B12 deficiency

This is a potential adverse effect of longer-term treatment (Liu et al., 2014; Niafar et al., 2015) and is not rare. It occurs in 10 to 30% of persons taking metformin. While usually these decreases in vitamin B12 are not serious (Kirpichnikov et al., 2002), in a few patients they may be. In patients with diabetes, metformin use has been associated not only with B12 deficiency but also with neuropathy.

We should:

1. Maybe check the vitamin B12 level at baseline?

2. Ask the person to take a multivitamin daily. Even though it is a problem with absorption, it may be overcome, in part, by increasing intake. Taking a multivitamin has been associated with a lower risk of low or borderline vitamin B12 in persons taking metformin (Kancherla et al., 2016).

3. Make sure the person is taking enough calcium. The absorption of vitamin B12 bound to intrinsic factor is a calcium-dependent process. Given calcium carbonate 1200 mg/day was reported to reverse the effect of metformin on vitamin B12 levels (Baumann et al., 2000). I would only recommend calcium supplements to those who have low calcium intake and should increase their calcium intake anyway.

4. Check the vitamin B12 level once a year (Andrade, 2016). One study in diabetic patients showed that vitamin B12 levels were checked in only about one-thirds of patients on long-term metformin treatment.

5. If the vitamin B12 level becomes clearly low, oral supplementation may not be good enough. We can treat this vitamin B12 deficiency by giving intramuscular hydroxocobalamin. Andrade (2016) has argued that currently available vitamin B12 levels can be inaccurate, are expensive, and may not be the best measure of clinical B12 deficiency. He, therefore, suggests that all patients treated with metformin simply get an injection of 1 mg of vitamin B12 once a year.

6. However, taking sublingual methylcobalamin every day has been shown to be as effective as an intramuscular injection of vitamin B12 (Parry-Strong et al., 2016) and is, obviously, more convenient. The dose is 1 mg/day. Yes, this is not a typo. The intramuscular dose is 1 mg per year but the sublingual dose is 1 mg per day.

NatureMade is a good brand for vitamins. It is made by the consumer division of Otsuka Pharmaceuticals. A dietician colleague told me that Solgar® is another good brand.

Lactic acidosis

Lactic acidosis is a very serious adverse effect that can occur with metformin. It is associated with 30 to 50% mortality. In the US, metformin carries a boxed warning ("black box warning") about the possibility of lactic acidosis.

Fortunately, lactic acidosis is very rare with metformin and it almost always occurs in persons with significant risk factors (discussed below). So, it is very important to not give metformin to persons with the following risk factors for lactic acidosis:

1. Age > 80 years.

The Prescribing Information states that metformin should not be started in persons 80 years or older unless measurement of creatinine clearance demonstrates that renal function is not reduced.

2. Heavy alcohol use. Either acute or chronic intake of large amounts of alcohol can potentiate the effect of metformin on lactate metabolism (Kirpichnikov et al., 2002).

3. Liver dysfunction (clinical or on laboratory testing)

4. Renal impairment.

Metformin should not be given to persons whose serum creatinine is greater than 1.5 mg/dL or whose estimated GFR is below 30 mL/min/1.73 m² (Andrade, 2016).

Also, if radiocontrast or general anesthesia is given, renal function may temporarily worsen, so metformin should be stopped temporarily in such situations (Kirpichnikov et al., 2002).

In elderly persons with lower lean body mass, use the estimated GFR rather than the serum creatinine, which may not be elevated in these persons even when the GFR is decreased (Kirpichnikov et al., 2002).

5. Current heart failure

6. Current hypoxia (Kirpichnikov et al., 2002)

7. Current significant infection (Kirpichnikov et al., 2002)

8. Use of topiramate along with metformin

Tips on prescribing metformin

Before we start

1. Counsel the patient regularly regarding diet and exercise. However, don't wait too long hoping that diet and exercise will be sufficient.

2. Think about metformin relatively early on in the course of the illness and antipsychotic treatment, before the metabolic adverse effects have become chronic. If other measures work, the metformin can always be reduced or stopped later.

3. Check for contraindications as discussed under Potential adverse effects of metformin.

4. Check hepatic function tests and estimated GFR (calculated from serum creatinine) because metformin is contraindicated in the presence of

liver or renal impairment.

5. Do a baseline assessment in order to help assess any progress. Check weight, abdominal circumference, hemoglobin A1C, and serum lipids.

Starting metformin

1. Counsel the patient to avoid heavy alcohol use.

2. Only prescribe metformin extended-release since it has fewer gastrointestinal adverse effects than immediate-release metformin.

3. Start with metformin XR 500 mg once a day. To reduce gastrointestinal adverse effects, this should be taken with the largest meal of the day for that particular person.

Titrating up

Metformin XR is available in the US as 500 mg, 850 mg, and 1000 mg pills.

1. Increase the dose by 500 mg/day every one to two weeks.

2. If possible, increase to the maximum dose of 2000 mg/day in a single dose or divided into two doses.

2. Topiramate

As discussed above, metformin may be used for metabolic syndrome associated with use of second-generation antipsychotics. Surprisingly, I have seen many more patients who had been prescribed topiramate for this purpose rather than metformin.

Does topiramate work?

A meta-analysis of eight randomized controlled clinical trials with 336 participants found that topiramate works to reduce weight gain associated with antipsychotic medications (Mahmood et al., 2013).

Topiramate may lead to weight loss in persons who are overweight or obese due to reasons other than being on a second-generation antipsychotic

(Mahmood et al., 2013).

Note: The use of topiramate to prevent or treat weight gain is not FDA-approved.

How well did it work?

The mean decrease in weight was – 6.2 lbs

Which means that many of the patients lost more than 6.2 lbs.

At what dose?

The dose of topiramate used for this purpose in clinical trials ranged from 100 mg/day to 300 mg/day.

But, because the side effects of topiramate may be quite significant at higher doses, we should try 100 or 150 mg for many weeks before considering higher doses.

Metformin or topiramate?

For antipsychotic-induced weight gain, metformin and topiramate lead to approximately the same amount of weight loss. But metformin should usually be preferred over topiramate because topiramate can be associated with (Ellinger et al., 2010):

– cognitive dulling

– risk of kidney stones

– more drug interactions, and

– adverse effects including psychiatric adverse effects.

Metformin AND topiramate for metabolic adverse effects?

Metformin and topiramate are two of the leading pharmacological options for treating metabolic syndrome associated with second-generation antipsychotic medications. Can they also be used together?

Is the combination more effective?

I am unaware of any study comparing the combination of metformin and topiramate to either of these medications alone.

But, this may be the case because in obese diabetic patients who were already on metformin, addition of topiramate led to a decrease in weight (Toplak et al., 2007). In this study, the mean dose of metformin was 1360 mg/day. At the end of the study, 24 weeks after topiramate was added to the metformin, average weight loss was 4.5% in patients receiving topiramate 96 mg/day, 6.5% in those receiving topiramate 192 mg/day, and 1.7% in those receiving placebo.

Similarly, one case report described a patient in which this metformin, ranitidine, and topiramate were used together to treat clozapine-induced weight gain (Greg Deardorff et al., 2014).

Potential problem with the combination

It is recommended that metformin and topiramate should not be used together. Why? Because they can both cause lactic acidosis, a very dangerous side effect, and the effect is additive.

The Prescribing Information for metformin includes in its Boxed Warning: "Risk factors for metformin-associated lactic acidosis include renal impairment, concomitant use of certain drugs (e.g. carbonic anhydrase inhibitors such as topiramate)...."

It also notes:

"Topiramate or other carbonic anhydrase inhibitors...frequently cause a decrease in serum bicarbonate and induce non-anion gap, hyperchloremic metabolic acidosis. Concomitant use of these drugs with GLUCOPHAGE or GLUCOPHAGE XR may increase the risk for lactic acidosis. Consider more frequent monitoring of these patients."

In the clinical trial discussed above (Toplak et al., 2007), while serum bicarbonate decreased slightly in those who received topiramate, there were no cases of clinically relevant metabolic acidosis.

Change in medication levels

A much less important issue is that if this combination is used, we should keep in mind that that metformin and topiramate can affect each other's levels (Manitpisitkul et al., 2014). When these two medications were used together, the metformin level increased and the topiramate level decreased.

But, the Prescribing Information for topiramate notes that topiramate was given along with metformin, the exposure to metformin (AUC) increased by 25% and the clearance of topiramate was decreased as well.

Bottom line

The treatment of obesity, especially in diabetic patients, is very important. While metformin and topiramate can be used together, we should be aware that this combination increases the risk of metabolic acidosis. So, the combination should be avoided unless essential.

If these medications are used together, it should preferably be done by or in consultation with a clinician who is able to monitor the patient for possible lactic acidosis including clinically and by laboratory tests.

Add aripiprazole to treat clozapine-induced weight gain?

Question: Patient has a marked increase in appetite and weight on clozapine. Metformin and topiramate were not tolerated. Numerous attempts were made to switch him to other antipsychotics or to decrease his clozapine dose, but his psychotic symptoms would worsen. What are the treatment options?

Clozapine is an invaluable treatment for persons with schizophrenia because it is effective in some of these patients even when other antipsychotics have not worked—so-called "treatment-resistant schizophrenia". This is why it is not usually possible to replace it with another medication. So, being able to effectively manage its side effects is absolutely essential.

Does it work?

Multiple systematic reviews and meta-analyses on this topic all agree among the few treatments shown to be effective for clozapine-induced weight gain is the addition of aripiprazole (Zimbron et al., 2016; Whitney et al., 2015; Choi et al., 2015).

Two randomized clinical trials: This is supported by one large (Fleischacker et al., 2010) and one small (Fan et al., 2013) randomized, double-blind, placebo-controlled clinical trial.

Supportive evidence: The addition of aripiprazole to clozapine was also effective in a small, open-label clinical trial (Henderson et al., 2006). Also, when added to olanzapine, aripiprazole was found to counteract olanzapine-induced increased appetite in rats (Snigdha et al., 2008).

Bottom line: All the evidence points in the same direction—that addition of aripiprazole to clozapine leads to weight loss.

How much weight loss?

We noted above that the addition of aripiprazole has been shown to be effective for clozapine-induced weight loss. But, this does not mean that it is a silver bullet. The amount of weight lost after the addition of aripiprazole varies from person to person, but we would like to get at least get some idea about how much benefit we can expect. After 16 weeks of treatment, the mean weight loss in the group in which aripiprazole was added to clozapine was about 4.7 lbs more than in the group in which placebo was added (Fleischacker et al., 2010).

A 5-pound weight loss is not a lot, BUT:

1. Clinical experience suggests that, for reasons that are not known, the weight loss from adding aripiprazole varies a lot from person to person. While the *average* weight loss is about 5 lbs, many patients lose more weight than this.

2. In addition to adding aripiprazole, it is important that some other non-pharmacological and/or pharmacological measures should also be considered simultaneously. This is because each intervention may have a modest effect but the effects may add up. The first-line option for clozapine-induced weight gain should probably be the addition of metformin. The addition of aripiprazole may be considered if metformin does not work adequately or is not tolerated.

3. If there is some weight loss in the first few months after the addition of aripiprazole, it is not clear how likely it is that over a longer duration of treatment it may slowly lead to greater weight loss.

4. Another reason to consider adding aripiprazole to clozapine is that it led not only to weight loss but to other metabolic benefits as well.

Adding aripiprazole has other metabolic benefits too

Fleischacker et al. (2010): Patients in whom aripiprazole was added to the clozapine had a greater decrease in body weight, body mass index (BMI), waist circumference, total cholesterol, and LDL cholesterol.

Fan et al. (2013): Those in whom aripiprazole was added to clozapine had a greater reduction in total body mass, lean body mass, and LDL cholesterol, and a greater improvement in glucose tolerance.

What about the illness?

Occasional case reports of worsening when aripiprazole was added to another antipsychotic have been published (Takeuchi and Remington, 2013). So, is this a concern when aripiprazole is added to clozapine?

In both of the studies discussed above, the severity of psychotic symptoms was systematically monitored using a standard rating scale (Fan et al., 2013; Fleischacker et al., 2010).

In one of them, the total score on the rating scale for psychosis (PANSS) decreased in both the aripiprazole and placebo groups (Fan et al., 2013). There were no serious adverse events in this study and there is no mention of psychosis worsening in any patients (Fan et al., 2013).

In the other study, similar numbers of patients in both groups (7% on placebo and 9% on aripiprazole) showed 30% or more improvement in the psychosis (Fleischacker et al., 2010).

These data are somewhat reassuring. But, it is possible that individual patients may worsen. In one study, of 108 patients in whom aripiprazole was added, two patients were reported to have had worsening (described as "severe psychotic disorder' and "severe auditory hallucinations") that were considered to be "possibly related" to the treatment (Fleischacker et al., 2010).

In individual patients, the addition of aripiprazole to clozapine can *sometimes* allow for a reduction in the dose of clozapine (Karunakaran et al., 2007). This is also borne out by clinical experience.

How much aripiprazole?

The optimal dose of aripiprazole to be added to clozapine to treat clozapine-induced weight gain is not known. But, it is probably not just a low dose like about 5 mg/day. The dose of aripiprazole added to clozapine was 15 mg/day in one study (Fan et al., 2013) and 5 to 15 mg/day (mean dose 11 mg/day) in the other (Fleischacker et al., 2010).

Add aripiprazole to olanzapine?

Note that we are *not* talking here about *switching* from olanzapine to aripiprazole; of course, that leads to weight loss. That's no surprise.

But, a randomized, double-blind, placebo-controlled clinical trial found that the addition of aripiprazole 15 mg/day reduced weight and BMI in overweight and obese patients who *continued to be on a stable dose of olanzapine* (Henderson et al., 2009).

As an extreme example, a case was published of a patient who was changed from high dose olanzapine plus amisulpride to high dose olanzapine plus aripiprazole and lost 37 pounds over four months without any other apparent reason for the weight loss (Boland and Chhabra, 2019).

What is the mechanism?

What is the mechanism by which aripiprazole helps reverse olanzapine-induced weight gain? This is easy to answer—the mechanism is not known (Deng et al., 2010).

References: See https://simpleandpractical.com/side-effects-references

CHAPTER 19: OTHER SIDE EFFECTS

EDEMA

Edema is a potential adverse effect of hydrazine MAO inhibitors like phenelzine and isocarboxazid.

It has been known for a long time (e.g., Dunleavy, 1977).

I have long used the mnemonic "Oh WISE" for some of the common side effects of MAOI. It stands for **O**rthostatic **H**ypotension, **W**eight gain, **I**nsomnia, **S**exual dysfunction, and **E**dema.

What to do?

There is no easy answer except to try elevation of feet,

1. Consider switching to tranylcypromine.

The edema may be due to interference with vitamin B6 metabolism that occurs with the hydrazine MAOIs.

However, tranylcypromine is structurally unrelated and edema can occur with tranylcypromine as well (Sours, 1962).

2. Try vitamin B6?

YAWNING

What is excessive yawning?

Yawning is, of course, a normal phenomenon when a person is sleepy, tired, or bored. And, it can also occur in a variety of other situations. But, the biology of yawning is not fully understood.

The first thing to note about excessive yawning as a side effect is that when we say "excessive", we mean that it is not due to other reasons like being tired, sleepy, hungry, etc. Before we call it excessive yawning, we should ask about how well the person has slept and whether they are feeling tired. Yawning can also occur when a person is hungry or hypoglycemic (Béné et al., 2014) and we should ask about this as well. But, patients with medication-induced excessive yawning report the strange experience of yawning over and over again even though deny feeling sleepy or tired.

Why does it matter?

Now, we may immediately ask—who cares? I guess the main reason the patient cares is that yawning repeatedly is embarrassing in social situations because it is seen as being rude or as a sign of being bored with the conversation. The symptoms can be so embarrassing or otherwise bothersome that patients in whom it is severe may be unwilling to continue on the medication. For example, in one case report, the person with antidepressant-induced yawning was himself a physician and his patients commented about his yawning, which bothered him so much that he discontinued the antidepressant (Beale and Murhphree, 2000). Similarly, in another case report, the patient found yawning episodes that occurred in the presence of clients and co-workers to be very distressing, and frequent comments about this from her husband were so bothersome that she asked for the dose of the medication to be reduced (Gutiérrez-Alvarez, 2007).

Also, persistent and excessive yawning can sometimes lead to facial or jaw pain and, occasionally, can even lead to dislocation of the lower jaw (e.g., Pae et al., 2003; Tesfaye et al., 1991; Tesfaye and Lal, 1990).

Medications and excessive yawning

SSRIs can be associated with excessive yawning and many case reports of this have been published (e.g., Roncero et al., 2013; Uher et al., 2009; Pal and Padala, 2009; Gutiérrez-Alvarez, 2007; Harada, 2006; Beale and Murphree, 2000). I have also definitely seen patients with this side effect.

On simpleandpractical.com, we have considered adverse events that were reported by patients in clinical trials as having occurred after the medication was started ("treatment-emergent adverse events") as presumably being side effects of the medication if they occurred at least twice as often as on placebo. See https://simpleandpractical.com/aehandouts for handouts listing such side effects for each psychotropic medication.

In those handouts, we see that "yawning" is noted as having been reported by 2% each of patients on citalopram, duloxetine, fluoxetine, and paroxetine. But, since I know a bit about how side effects are identified in clinical trials, I doubt that they checked to make sure that the yawning was not related to somnolence. Also in clinical trials, they don't specifically ask about specific side effects. So, in my opinion, the actual incidence of excessive yawning with various antidepressants and with other medications is not known.

Excessive yawning has been reported not only with SSRIs but also with other classes of antidepressants— SNRIs (e.g., Chen and Lu, 2009; De Las Cuevas and Sanz, 2007) and tricyclic antidepressants (e.g., Goldberg, 1983-84).

While other psychotropic and non-psychotropic medications can be also associated with excessive yawning, antidepressants are probably the class of medications that are most likely to cause it (Patatanian et al., 2011).

Excessive yawning can also be found in many neurological conditions including migraine, epilepsy, stroke, etc. (Teive et al., 2018; Walusinski, 2009).

[Optional to read: At least two case reports of excessive yawning associated with methylphenidate have been published (Gallup and Gallup, 2020; Naguy et al., 2019)]

Management of antidepressant-induced excessive yawning

An important thing is to realize that it is due to the antidepressant! Case reports have described how patients were referred for neurological or other evaluations because at first it was not realized that the excessive yawning was due o the antidepressant (e.g., Pal and Padala, 2009).

In most cases of antidepressant-induced excessive yawning, nothing needs to be done except to reassure the patient. But, if the excessive yawning is frequent and persists, it can be quite distressing to the patient.

1. If other neurological symptoms, including migraine, are present, the patient should be referred to a neurologist for evaluation.

2. Like most, but not all, side effects, antidepressant-induced excessive yawning is typically dose-dependent (Roncero et al., 2013; Patatanian et al., 2011). So, dose reduction can be tried if that is clinically feasible. In many

of the published case reports, the excessive yawning improved as the dose was reduced (Patatanian et al., 2011) and in many cases, it goes away completely on a reduced dose of the antidepressant (Roncero et al., 2013; Gutiérrez-Alvarez, 2007).

3. If possible, switching to another class of medication, may result in improvement or even resolution of this side effect.

4. I could not find any published case of bupropion causing excessive yawning. Also, case reports have been published where a patient who had excessive sweating on an SSRI was switched to bupropion and the side effect went away (e.g., Nazar et al., 2015; Beale and Murphree, 2000).

5. A case report was published describing the successful treatment of antidepressant-induced excessive yawning by the addition of cyproheptadine 4 mg three times a day. But, my concern about this is that regular use of cyproheptadine could also antagonize the beneficial effect of the medication (Hollander et al., 1992; Feder, 1991; Goldbloom and Kennedy, 1991), although this did not happen in that case report where it was used to treat anorgasmia and excessive yawning (Cohen, 1992).

References: See https://simpleandpractical.com/side-effects-references

ABOUT THE AUTHOR

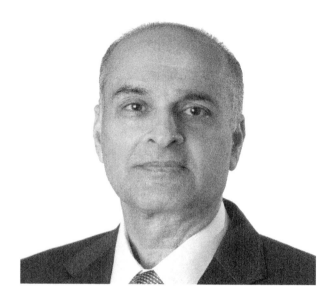

Dr. Rajnish ("Raj") Mago, MD, is a psychiatrist in Philadelphia who treats patients with mood disorders, anxiety disorders, and adult ADHD. For over 25 years, he has treated a large number of patients, including those who were difficult-to-treat. His research has focused on the assessment, prediction, and treatment of side effects of psychotropic medications and on the development of newer medications. Dr. Mago has been widely recognized for his teaching ability and for his "Simple and Practical" approach to learning. He has received a number of awards for his teaching and other contributions to the field. He is the Founder and Editor-in-Chief of *Simple and Practical Medical Education* (simpleandpractical.com), a website devoted to providing the most clinically useful education in the simplest, briefest, and most convenient manner possible.

Printed in Great Britain
by Amazon

61038817R00208